MW00336917

A Call to Action

A Call to Action

First Edition

Library of Congress Cataloging-in-Publication Data

Moore, Geoffrey E.
    A Call to Action: the story of the Prostate Cancer Foundation
    Includes index.
    Library of Congress Control Number: 2004092506
    ISBN 0-9646425-2-2
    1. Prostate Cancer Foundation—History. 2. Health I. Title.

The *Time* magazine cover reproduced on page 39 is used with
permission from Time Life Pictures/Getty Images. FORTUNE is a
registered trademark of *Fortune* magazine, a division of Time Inc. The
photograph of Rupert Murdoch and Michael Milken on page 127 is
provided by and used with the permission of *The Los Angeles Times.*
The Ken Griffey Jr. photograph on page 128 is provided by and used
with the permission of Tom DiPace.

The paper used in this publication meets the requirements of the
National Information Standards Organization (NISO).

Printed in the United States of America

For the first time in history, patients diagnosed with diseases that used to be fatal have a realistic hope that cures will emerge in their lifetimes.

This book is dedicated to everyone who is working to make that hope a reality.

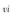

Contents

"History will show that the field of prostate cancer research bloomed when the Prostate Cancer Foundation began. They've done more than any other organization to reduce deaths."

Patrick Walsh, M.D.
Chairman, Clinical Faculty
Brady Urological Institute, Johns Hopkins University
Author, "Dr. Patrick Walsh's Guide to Surviving Prostate Cancer"

"Mike Milken has changed everything by bringing business discipline to the field. Lots of people write checks; but nobody changed the culture until he came along."

Stuart Holden, M.D.
Medical Director, Louis Warshaw Prostate Cancer Center at Cedars-Sinai Medical Center
Medical Director, The Prostate Cancer Foundation

"Remember that old Archimedes principle that if you give me a lever long enough, I can lift the world? The Prostate Cancer Foundation has been the ultimate lever for progress."

Jonathan Simons, M.D.
Director, Winship Cancer Institute, Emory University

"I cannot tell you what a difference the Prostate Cancer Foundation has made – I'm just blown away by what has been accomplished. For the first time in my long career, I believe that major victories over cancer are coming – they really are. There are many people alive around the world today because of Mike Milken's work."

Donald Coffey, Ph.D.
Former President, American Association for Cancer Research
Director of Urological Research,
Johns Hopkins University School of Medicine

Introduction

*I*n the grand sweep of history, it wasn't long ago that many human diseases were assumed to be the consequence of "bad air." Whatever was causing disease didn't just *live* in the air – it was believed to be created by the air itself. According to this theory of spontaneous generation, if maggots appeared on fetid meat, that was seen as evidence that the meat, which was dead, created the living bugs. Following this logic, if a human patient developed a fever, the cause was his own failing flesh or weak blood. Without an understanding that infectious agents had invaded the body, there was no point in trying to control their transmission.

It took 250 years, from van Leeuwenhoek's invention of the first practical microscope in the 1670s to Fleming's discovery of penicillin in the 1920s, for the complete development of the germ theory of disease. Along the way, Pasteur demolished the idea of spontaneous generation of microorganisms, Semmelweis demonstrated that childbed fever could be controlled if doctors and midwives simply washed their hands, and Lister made surgery safer by applying antiseptic chemicals. Yet, as recently as 1900, one of every five children born in the U.S. didn't live to celebrate a fifth birthday. In the general population, tuberculosis, pneumonia and

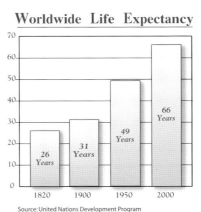

Worldwide Life Expectancy

Source: United Nations Development Program

diarrhea caused more than half of all deaths. Life expectancy was 50 years in the U.S., only 31 worldwide.

During the 20th century, the global lifespan gap narrowed as modernizing communication and transportation brought information, training and caregivers to what we now call the developing world. Life expectancy increased 54 percent to 77 years in the U.S. and more than doubled to 66 years worldwide. Improvements in basic sanitation, antisepsis and infection control had combined with the development of antibiotics and vaccines to extend lives. It was arguably one of the greatest achievements in history.

(There have been setbacks – AIDS, hemorrhagic fever outbreaks, SARS, the rise of other antibiotic-resistant infections – but their effects on the general population to date have not had a major effect on average life spans.)

Following World War II, medical researchers increasingly turned their attention to what had emerged as the great modern killers: heart disease and cancer. Although there is some controversy about whether infectious agents might be involved in the pre-symptomatic stage of these diseases, the current consensus holds that they develop from a confluence of genes, lifestyle and age. What we know for sure is that they are deadly. More than half of us are expected to die from cardiovascular disease or some form of cancer.

Deaths from cardiovascular illnesses have declined steadily over the past 40 years because of better treatments and prevention. Progress against cancer has been slower, largely because of our limited knowledge of its cellular basis. Most treatments still involve cutting, burning or poisoning tumors. But recent advances in molecular biology, genetics and information systems have vastly increased our understanding of cancer's *mechanisms* – how it starts and spreads through the body. That offers real hope that we will be able to predict and forestall its onset or treat its symptoms as dramatically as vaccines and antibiotics dealt with infection.

One of every two American men and one of every three women are diagnosed with cancer at some time in their lives. Many others die from different causes with undiagnosed cancers growing in their bodies. Future progress against heart disease, stroke, AIDS, diabetes and other killers will extend lives to the point where more of these hidden cancers will develop into symptomatic disease. That makes the information in this book especially relevant and important. Although it tells the story of the Prostate Cancer Foundation (PCF), it also suggests a broad approach to medical research that could lead to better treatments and faster cures for many illnesses that are likely to affect you or your family.

That approach has already produced the impressive research progress described in Chapter 12. But as other chapters in this book explain, it has also changed the *process* of medical research by creating a new model for interaction across the boundaries of academia, industry, government and foundations. As this book was about to go to press, the National Cancer Institute (NCI) convened a remarkable Washington, D.C. "Leadership Roundtable" that brought executives from several of America's largest corporations together with the nation's leading cancer experts to develop new strategies based on just such interaction. The PCF's president and chairman both participated in developing what the NCI's Director called "the Roundtable's wealth of substantive solutions" (see Chapter 14).

It is a testament to the brilliant concept and execution of the PCF mission that this organization, which had been no more than an idea 11 years earlier, would have such a profound impact on national cancer policy. The PCF had helped to make the medical research process increasingly efficient and effective by attracting more of the best and brightest scientific and medical graduates to research careers. More than many charitable organizations, the PCF recognized that the political, financial and cultural components of research programs affect the prospects of success as much as the technical skills of the researchers.

The PCF approach differs somewhat from that of traditional funders like the Rockefeller Foundation, which spurred massive improvements in public health a century ago, or the Gates Foundation, which today is saving lives by devoting much of its resources to known strategies of prevention and treatment in developing nations. The PCF not only funds research on improved treatments and cures not yet available; it also seeks to remove roadblocks to the development of such advances. Founded in 1993 as "CaP CURE," the PCF started with three goals:

1. A substantial increase in the human, social and financial resources devoted to research on all serious diseases;
2. Greater focus on reducing the burden of cancer in its many forms;
3. Significant growth in programs to deal with the specific problem of prostate cancer.

The first goal recognized that the greatest benefit to society would be achieved by increasing the share of the economy devoted to funding medical research on all deadly diseases. CaP CURE would not play the zero-sum game – a practice of diverting money from one disease to fund research in another area – preferring to increase funding for all diseases. It would encourage teamwork among the many disease-advocacy organizations and seek to expand resources for everyone, especially through budget increases for the National Institutes of Health and for regional centers of medical excellence.

Second, within the subset of diseases we call cancer, most medical experts agree that progress against one type of cancer usually leads to improved treatments for other types. Thus, for example, new chemotherapeutic agents shown to be effective in treating breast cancer are now being tested against cancers of the prostate, colon and other organs. Similar cross-disease synergies are found in the areas of surgical techniques, adjuvant hormonal therapy, radiation treatment, gene therapy, nutritional interventions and other lifestyle changes.

CaP CURE's third goal was to raise the profile of prostate cancer in terms of the number of researchers working on it, the funds devoted to it, and awareness of it among the growing cohort of men most at risk. Back in 1993, few people knew that this disease affects one of every six men in America. Even fewer knew that the problem was expected to get worse as the baby-boom generation grew older.

The name "CaP CURE" was created in an attempt to reflect these three goals. "Ca" is a shorthand notation that medical professionals often use to designate cancer; "CaP" indicates cancer of the prostate; and "CURE" symbolized the ultimate goal of major progress against all deadly diseases.

Over the past decade, CaP CURE participated in several activities, chronicled in this book, that advanced broad programs of medical research: the National Cancer Summit; the Working Meeting on Standards at the Food and Drug Administration; the March on Washington by 600 cancer organizations; new medical research initiatives at the Department of Defense; greater interaction between for-profit companies and non-profit institutions; and more. These programs went a long way toward meeting the first two goals.

While the research funded by CaP CURE has focused primarily on prostate cancer, it has also been successful in helping to focus public policy on the need to increase resources for all medical research – government and private funding has grown to several times the 1993 level – and to increase focus on the medical infrastructure. These achievements, along with the establishment of FasterCures / The Center for Accelerating Medical Solutions, the National Dialogue on Cancer (which recently became C-Change: Collaborating to Conquer Cancer) and other groups, will allow CaP CURE to concentrate most of its efforts on its third goal. So early in 2003, a decade after its launch, CaP CURE changed its name to the Prostate Cancer Foundation. CaP CURE had long been the world's largest philanthropic source of funds for prostate cancer research. Now it has a name that will more effectively build awareness of its mission.

Throughout this book, most references to "CaP CURE," even in direct quotations, have been changed to the Prostate Cancer Foundation or "PCF."

Foreword

Andrew von Eschenbach, M.D.

$\mathscr{L}$ife is filled with interesting and sometimes poignant coincidences. Thirty years ago, I had not yet met Mike Milken. But our lives were to follow parallel tracks that would eventually bring us together in the national effort to advance medical science. Both of us were close to our fathers, who had a profound influence on our lives. Both of our fathers were diagnosed with cancer in the early 1970s. In the mid-1970s, Mike and I both learned that our fathers' cancers had spread, leaving a

President Bush named Andrew von Eschenbach to head the National Cancer Institute in 2001. Dr. von Eschenbach is a nationally known urologic surgeon who previously led the Genitourinary Cancer Center at the University of Texas M. D. Anderson Cancer Center, where he also served as Executive Vice President and Chief Academic Officer and Director of the Prostate Cancer Research Program. A founding member of C-Change: Collaborating to Conquer Cancer, he was president-elect of the American Cancer Society at the time of his appointment to the NCI, where he is the 12th director since the Institute's establishment in 1938.

poor prognosis. We each took our fathers to distant cancer centers in search of a better outcome. Before they died (at the end of the '70s), we each rededicated ourselves to a lifetime of searching for medical solutions – Mike through what has been more than a quarter century of remarkable philanthropy, and I through medical research, clinical practice and, now, public service.

Mike and I have much in common. We each have prostate cancer, and in both cases the disease is in remission. Each of us has children to whom we want to leave a legacy of progress against disease. We are both blessed with devoted wives who have encouraged us at every stage of our careers.

When Mike and I initially met, it was through a mutual friend, Dr. Neal Kassell, a prominent neurosurgeon. Neal had been a medical student at the University of Pennsylvania when he first met Mike, who was then a graduate student at the University's Wharton School of Business. Neal and I were later colleagues as we completed our post-graduate medical training.

One Sunday in 1993, Neal called me at home to describe the case of a friend whose prostate cancer profile seemed to match those of a group of patients I was studying at the M.D. Anderson Cancer Center in Houston. He asked if this patient, then unnamed, but later identified as Mike Milken, could call me. When Mike and I spoke later that day, I invited him to join me in Houston, where a conference of leading prostate-cancer specialists was about to begin. Within weeks after meeting these doctors, Mike established the Prostate Cancer Foundation (PCF), originally known as CaP CURE. This book documents the PCF's amazing impact. It is an inspiring primer for anyone setting out to change the course of history.

Mike had been supporting medical research on many diseases through a different organization, the Milken Family Foundation, for many years before he was diagnosed with advanced prostate cancer. But it wasn't until he began an intensive study of the prostate cancer field that he realized the research process was flawed. I consider it both genius and grace that he recognized it would take more than money to fix this process. It would require fundamental changes in the way the community of medical and scientific investigators goes about its work.

One of the major problems was that specialists like surgeons, medical oncologists, radiologists, biomedical researchers and other scientists had too little communication outside their respective specialties. This limited research progress and tended to deny patients the kind of fully integrated treatment plans they deserve. Another concern was that researchers were spending far too much time writing applications for grants and were not being held fully accountable for how those grants were used. Finally, not nearly enough of the brightest young scientists and physicians were entering research careers.

The Prostate Cancer Foundation has transformed the field by addressing each of these issues with uncommon creativity. First, it told researchers to send their most important ideas that had not been funded, to keep the applications short, and to stop wasting time looking backward by documenting their previous achievements. This made the process of obtaining a research grant faster and easier. But there was a string attached – a brilliant string. Each year, all grant recipients around the world were to attend the PCF's Scientific Retreat, where they would be required to share their research with other institutions and with specialists in other fields.

This had a dramatic effect. The field of prostate cancer research, which had occupied a quiet corner of medicine, was suddenly energized with original and imaginative ideas. That in turn influenced the agency I now head to increase its commitment to prostate cancer. And that attracted new people into the field.

Another effect was an improvement in the quality of research reporting. I can personally attest that all of us then at M.D. Anderson prepared intensively for Prostate Cancer Foundation presentations. So did our counterparts at every other major medical center. We knew that our work would receive a rigorous multi-disciplinary, multi-institutional review and we'd better have it right.

The PCF Scientific Retreats also exposed us to the thinking of leaders in such other fields as business and public policy. It's quite an experience for a young doctor or scientist to find himself seated next to a U.S. Senator or a Fortune 500 CEO, not just because of the reflected glory, but because the thinking of these leaders tends to focus on *results*. More than a few medical researchers have returned from PCF meetings with a deeper understanding that their bright ideas do nothing to relieve the suffering of patients. The only thing that counts is the successful translation of those ideas into practical therapies.

When I began my medical career, most cancer researchers were looking for a "magic bullet" that could eliminate tumors. We now recognize that there is no magic bullet, but there can be an effective strategy based on the *integration* of various interventions. The Prostate Cancer Foundation has furthered this trend toward integration of both research and patient care. We now better understand that cancer is not about an abstract thing called a tumor so much as it is a disease process in an individual person. The Foundation has also supported important research that has moved the field toward more targeted interventions based on knowledge of the underlying mechanisms of cancer. Most of all, the PCF created a sense of urgency that has changed the culture of research.

Over the past decade, few people have done more to advance the fight against serious diseases than Mike Milken. His personal vision, energy and leadership of the Prostate Cancer Foundation have truly transformed the way we do research. His extraordinary access to leaders in diverse sectors of American society has helped bring new recognition to the importance of medical research and the dedicated people who carry it forward. He knows how critically important it is to accelerate the pace of progress because every day people are suffering and dying. That is why Mike has recently established a Washington-based think tank, FasterCures / The Center for Accelerating Medical Solutions, which aims to help shorten the path to improved treatment outcomes and eventual cures for all deadly diseases. May God continue to bless him, his family, and the work he does to improve the lives of people everywhere.

"Omigod!"

"*Based on his age, it seemed unlikely that he had prostate cancer. But I did a blood test and examined him. As soon as I felt his prostate, I knew instantly that he had cancer and that it had spread. After 20 years of practicing urology, you can tell just by the condition of the prostate even before it's confirmed by a biopsy. This was not some subtle indication; it was very obvious. Another thing 20 years of practice teaches you: Don't blurt out something like 'Oh my God!' You keep your cool.*"

There's nothing pretentious about Stuart Holden, M.D., even if he is one of America's most distinguished urologists. He's been called "Skip" his entire life. But his usually ebullient manner turns serious when he describes the most difficult part of his work – confirming the worst fears of worried patients that they have cancer. In the case of one of his most famous patients, Michael Milken, the task was compounded by the knowledge that Milken had just emerged from the devastating strain of a legal battle that had become one of the 20th century's most overwrought media events.

It was early 1993 and Mike Milken had just started to return to active leadership in educational and medical philanthropy, areas that he'd pursued intently since the 1970s. After going through hell and back, it was time to have some fun. For Milken, nothing was more fun than figuring out creative and effective ways to give back to society the wealth he had earned as Wall Street's most important financier since J. P. Morgan. [Details of Milken's career are at www.mikemilken.com.] First, though, he was overdue for a routine medical checkup.

"I saw a very fine internist," recalls Milken, *"and he did the usual poking and prodding. Then I told him I wanted a test for prostate cancer because my friend Steve Ross, the late chairman of Time Warner, had recently passed away from that disease. The doctor told me that at age 46, I was too young to worry about it. I think I said something like 'Humor me; I can afford it.' "*

The news started out bad for Milken and then just got worse. His first indication was the Prostate Specific Antigen (PSA) blood test, which prompts doctors to do further testing if it's elevated. The upper limit of the normal PSA range is 4 ng/ml. Milken's was 24. A friend who had been treated for prostate cancer recommended Skip Holden, a specialist at Cedars-Sinai Medical Center in Los Angeles. Holden performed a digital rectal exam and repeated the PSA, which showed the same elevated reading. Then he did a biopsy, which definitively confirmed the presence of prostate cancer. One evaluation from the biopsy – called the Gleason score – measures a cancer's aggressiveness. On a scale of 2 to 10, with 10 being the most aggressive, Milken's score was 9.

There was more bad news. Further tests showed cancer had spread to Milken's lymph nodes, which were grossly enlarged. At the time, the prognosis for a man with cancer that advanced was 12 to 18 months of life. Another leading specialist told Milken and his wife, Lori, to get their affairs in order and seek psychological counseling to deal with the fact that his disease was terminal.

When Skip Holden told Milken just how grave the situation appeared, he expected the usual emotional response from a patient who has been handed a virtual death sentence. Instead …

"Mike was outwardly passive. But I could see the wheels turning as soon as he absorbed the blow. He was almost immediately in crisis-management mode. Within minutes, he had gathered every detail of my contact information including my home phone number. That night, I was on conference calls with him to several top medical scientists around the country, some of whom he knew from his earlier support of medical research

through the Milken Family Foundation. He was quickly spreading the net."

What happened next – and continues to this day – helps explain why tens of thousands of American men who were expected to be in their graves are walking around today. Over the decade beginning in 1993, actual prostate cancer mortality has been driven down, not up as the experts projected. This book tells the story of the organization that was born from Milken's personal ordeal as "CaP CURE" and is now called the Prostate Cancer Foundation.

Cancer was nothing new

Several of Milken's close relatives, including his father, had succumbed to various forms of cancer. But none was as young as he was at the time of diagnosis. As early as 1972, when his mother-in-law was diagnosed with breast cancer, Milken had begun a quest for medical solutions through a combination of study, involvement with the medical community and philanthropy. After his father died from melanoma in 1979, he joined with his brother Lowell and their families to formalize their efforts in a charitable organization. The result was the Milken Family Foundation, which opened its doors early in 1982. (Lowell Milken is a business executive and educational pioneer as well as a major philanthropist, both through the Milken Family Foundation and through the L&S Milken Foundation, a private charity that he heads with his wife, Sandy.)

From the beginning, Mike Milken was determined to help brilliant young medical investigators early in their careers. During the 1970s, he had traveled to leading medical centers around the country, originally in an effort to help his dying father. Later, he met with medical school deans and prominent physicians who deepened his understanding of the gap between the promise and the reality of medical research. One of the many things he learned was that the best young research physicians were too often tempted to leave their low-paying jobs at the laboratory bench to pursue more-lucrative clinical practices treating patients.

As Milken talked to young doctors and scientists in the 1980s, he was impressed with their dedication and convinced that most hadn't entered medicine to get rich. (That was consistent with Milken's long experience financing emerging entrepreneurs. He points out that virtually every truly successful business leader he worked with in his financial career started out with a plan to accomplish something and create value. The personal financial rewards they later enjoyed were a by-product, not the original motivation.) But these young medical scientists did have to feed their growing families, save for their children's education and plan for retirement. So Milken decided to establish a formal program – the Milken Family Foundation Cancer Research Awards – that would allow some of these researchers to stay in their labs for a few more crucial years.

One friend who helped set up the Research Awards program was Samuel Broder, M.D., who later would become the Director of the National Cancer Institute, where his path would again cross with Milken's (see Chapter 3). "Of all the programs we've supported over the last generation," says Milken, "the biggest payoff in terms of social benefit has come from the awards to young investigators." Among those who received awards in the 1980s were Dr. Dennis Slamon, who later discovered Herceptin, a revolutionary break-through in the treatment of one type of breast cancer; Dr. Bert Vogelstein, who did pioneering work on the crucial p53 gene whose mutant form is believed to be involved in more than half of human cancers; Dr. Owen Witte, whose subsequent work provided the basis for the development of the breakthrough drug Gleevec, now used as a frontline therapy for patients with chronic myelogenous leukemia; Dr. Lawrence Einhorn, who as the developer of a highly successful chemotherapy regimen for testicular cancer, later treated five-time Tour de France winner Lance Armstrong; Dr. Philip Leder, a pioneer in molecular biology who contributed to the deci-phering of the genetic code; Dr. Charles Myers, who went on to become Chief of the Clinical Pharmacology branch of the National Cancer Institute and today heads the American Institute for Diseases of the Prostate; and many more.

After two decades of this kind of involvement, Milken acquired a deep layman's knowledge of cancer and other serious diseases. He could talk knowledgeably about breast cancer, melanoma, brain tumors, neurological disorders, AIDS, leukemia and more. That made it all the more surprising when he realized how little he knew about prostate cancer, the most common non-skin cancer in America. Even more shocking was the fact that little was being done about prostate cancer.

The conventional view at the time was that money wasn't available for prostate cancer research because there were no new ideas. Researchers responded that it was futile to spend months developing grant proposals that would be rejected for lack of funds. Milken decided to jump into the middle of this vicious circle and see if he could pull off something revolutionary. Something as revolutionary as the changes he had wrought in democratizing the capital markets beginning in the late 1960s when he figured out how to provide access to capital for entrepreneurs who had great ideas but little financial backing.

Typically, Milken didn't see things through the conventional lens. "The problem isn't a lack of financial capital," he said. "The scarce resource is human capital." He figured he'd better get working on changing that because he didn't have much time. And 35,000 American men expected to die from prostate cancer in 1993 shared his plight.

Where to Start?

*D*ealing with your own treatment plan is a full-time job for most cancer patients. But the more Milken studied his disease, the more he realized that treatment for its advanced forms was all too often ineffective. So he began to sketch out a three-part plan:

1. Stay alive long enough to make a difference.

2. Jump-start new programs in the field of prostate cancer that could offer hope to the millions of men who will face this disease in their lifetimes.

3. Create a better model for the way researchers "do science" that could accelerate solutions for all serious diseases.

It was incredibly ambitious. Skip Holden had told him that the field of prostate cancer research was moribund. Many of the best scientists avoided the field because money wasn't available. But Milken wouldn't hear of it. "If that's the case," he said, "we'll change it." Holden recalls his reaction:

> *"I was shocked by the chutzpah of Mike – one person, a layman, who thought he could pull this off and change the culture of how you do science. And change the dynamics of the National Cancer Institute. I was skeptical. But he had amazing creativity and energy. For example, he wanted multiple institutions to do collaborative projects. That was unheard of. He wanted to bring in the for-profit side. In those days, academic researchers considered any for-profit participation to be a taint on their academic purity. Mike also wanted to raise public awareness through various advocacy programs, something that hadn't been*

*done with prostate cancer. I was stimulated beyond belief. This
was something I'd wanted to do my whole career and I didn't
imagine it could be done. I was awestruck; but I still remained
skeptical."*

The challenge Milken wanted to take on was part of a quest the
medical infrastructure had been pursuing for a century. Congress
had established the first really organized approach to medical
research in the late 1800s when it created the agency that would
become the National Institutes of Health. In 1927, a bill authorized
"a reward for the discovery of a successful cure for cancer, and a
commission to inquire into and ascertain the success of such cure."
The reward was $5 million and the commission was the predecessor
of what became the National Cancer Institute (NCI) in 1938.

In 1971, President Richard Nixon called for a War on Cancer in
his State of the Union speech. *"The time has come,"* he said, *"when
the same kind of concentrated effort that split the atom and took man
to the moon should be turned toward conquering this dread disease. Let
us make a total national commitment to achieve this goal. America has
long been the wealthiest nation in the world. Now it is time we became
the healthiest nation in the world."* A few months later, Nixon signed
the National Cancer Act.

Reflecting on the 30th anniversary of the National Cancer Act in
the Journal of the American Medical Association, former NCI
Director Samuel Broder was blunt: *"At the time the Act was signed,
we had the most rudimentary knowledge of how cells were related, how
genes are coordinately expressed, how many things may go wrong at a
genetic or somatic level in the genome in various cancers – let alone how
to make them right, how to fix them. We hadn't the slightest clue."*

After decades of work, including massive strides to unlock the
human genome, hope was rising. The number of deaths caused by
several cancers had begun to decline slightly. But prospects for
breakthroughs in prostate cancer in 1993 were depressingly bleak.
The number of deaths was rising and was expected to rise even
faster toward the end of the century as the baby boomer generation reached the most vulnerable ages.

Worse still, not much was being done about it. At the time, government funding for prostate cancer research totaled about $250 per man diagnosed. That compared with more than $1,400 per breast cancer case and tens of thousands for every AIDS case. Lewis Sullivan, M.D., the former Secretary of Health and Human Services, noted that *"despite the record increase in new prostate cases, prostate cancer research remains significantly underfunded."* And virtually nothing was spent by states and localities.

Researchers at competing medical centers rarely shared their findings. Few of these centers had a well-developed program of prostate cancer research. There was little coordination of the few clinical trials in the field. Human tissue – tumors, skin and blood – was mostly unavailable to researchers. Not surprisingly, medical school graduates looking for resident fellowships were discouraged from pursuing prostate cancer specialties. One brilliant young doctor was told by his mentor that going into prostate cancer would be "career suicide" because there was no money for grants.

> *"In 1993, the NCI had spent all its money – a substantial amount of it on AIDS – and the last thing they wanted to hear was that there was another cancer out there that needed major funding,"* says Patrick Walsh, M.D., Chairman of the Brady Urological Institute at Johns Hopkins University. *"What I heard from the NCI was that prostate cancer wasn't important and there was no reason to put dollars into it. Nothing could have been further from the truth. But that was what they said. Whether they believed it, I don't know, but it was the excuse they gave for not emphasizing this cancer."*

Don't try to spell check it

At the time, there was little coordination of efforts between American cancer scientists and people doing research in other countries. Academic researchers had limited contact with their counterparts at pharmaceutical and biotechnology companies. And there weren't enough cross-specialty encounters among surgeons, oncologists, radiologists and other caregivers.

Several other problems hampered the field of prostate cancer back in 1993. For example, nutrition wasn't taken seriously enough to be considered "hard science" by most investigators. And public awareness was virtually non-existent. Prostate cancer was the subject of relatively few published articles or scientific papers. Many newspapers and magazines had never published an article about the disease. (As a hint of what's to come, the number of such articles in 2002 exceeded 20,000.)

Most public figures who were stricken with prostate cancer kept quiet about it. The disease was "in the closet," as breast cancer had been a generation earlier before people like Betty Ford and Happy Rockefeller spoke out. There were no well-known advocacy organizations for prostate cancer. Most people didn't even know how to pronounce the name of the disease. The word "prostate" was so uncommon that the spell-check feature of Microsoft Word corrected it to "prostrate."

On the political front, the Administration had proposed new legislation that threatened to impose unprecedented regulatory restrictions on the healthcare industry, which could affect research being conducted by biotechnology and pharmaceutical companies. As a result, these companies' stock prices plummeted by 50 percent. In response, the companies cut their research budgets.

With little research, there was little hope of progress in the treatment of prostate cancer. In fact, many experts doubted that any form of treatment improved survival, or whether it was even worthwhile to detect the cancer through the use of the PSA or the digital rectal exam. There was no doubt, however, about one fact: thousands of American men were dying from prostate cancer every month.

None of this did anything to cheer Mike Milken. As he began to analyze the situation, he realized it would take more than smart people and money to accelerate progress against cancer. He would have to change the process, modify the culture, redirect history.

Houston, We Have a Problem

*M*ilken's first chance to do something came in February 1993, only two weeks after his diagnosis. He had deferred the initiation of therapy until he could convince himself that he and Holden had figured out the best strategy. As part of his thorough study of the disease, he had been talking to several doctors around the country. One was Neal Kassell, an old friend who was a leading neurosurgeon at the University of Virginia. Kassell suggested that Milken see Andrew von Eschenbach, then the director of the Prostate Cancer Research Program at the University of Texas M.D. Anderson Cancer Center in Houston, who was studying a particular subset of prostate cancer patients similar to Milken. The cancer in these patients had spread to their lymph nodes, but had not invaded their bones.

A non-invasive scan of Milken's skeleton at Cedars-Sinai hadn't shown any bone involvement, but the only way to be sure was to test the bone marrow. Kassell said von Eschenbach was one of the best specialists to oversee that. "I'll call Andy and ask him to meet with you," he told Milken.

"I'll be happy to see you," von Eschenbach told Milken later that day, "but it's going to be kind of crazy around here this week because we're hosting a conference of prostate cancer specialists from many of the top cancer centers." Milken said he'd like to attend, a bold suggestion since the conference wasn't for patients, but von Eschenbach agreed when Milken said he'd bring his urologist, Skip Holden.

"It's funny that you should call me about that conference, Mike," said Holden later that afternoon. "I'm sitting here looking at the M.D. Anderson brochure describing it." They agreed it would be a good opportunity for Milken to learn more about the disease and meet many of the leading researchers and clinicians from around the country.

Because this was a professional meeting, Holden registered Milken as "Dr. Robert Hackel," using Milken's middle name and the surname of his father-in-law. Milken had already studied so much about the disease that he felt comfortable talking to the professionals. It gave him pause, however, when the experts showed graphic slides of tumors similar to his and talked about survival times measured in months.

"Mike took in all the information," recalls Holden. "I've never met anyone who could sort through and filter so much confusing data and distill it in his mind to the relevant points. Perhaps his experiences trading securities in real time – where numbers are flying at you constantly – helped train him for this."

It wasn't long before Milken disclosed his real identity and started to probe about the state of prostate cancer research. One of the speakers Milken approached was Donald Coffey, Ph.D., a truly remarkable man widely hailed as "the father of prostate cancer research in America." The holder of multiple professorships at The Johns Hopkins University, Coffey would later become president of the American Association for Cancer Research, whose membership includes 19,000 laboratory and clinical cancer researchers. His gentlemanly Southern accent and habit of performing magic tricks belie his commanding influence in medicine. He has mentored dozens of young scientists and physicians who have gone on to leadership positions at medical institutions nationwide. Coffey and other doctors Milken met in Houston told him there were lots of things they wanted to do, but there was little money available from the National Cancer Institute.

We're here to help

Within days, Holden was sitting with Milken in the office of Dr. Samuel Broder, then the Director of the National Cancer Institute at its sprawling campus in Bethesda, Maryland. *"Most doctors have no idea how Washington works, how the levers of power operate,"* says Holden. *"But Mike was completely comfortable in that environment. He didn't go hat in hand; he went as someone who was there to help the NCI get the money they needed from Congress."*

The conversation began with a review of the Milken Family Foundation's work in supporting medical research over the past decade, an effort in which Broder had been involved. Then Milken cut to the chase:

> *"There's not enough going on in prostate cancer, Sam,"* he told Broder. *"For 20 years, I thought I was doing everything I could for cancer – giving money, trying to identify the brightest young investigators, bringing in people like you to help with our awards. But it wasn't enough. I need to be more actively involved. Let's have a call to action and get Congress to focus on this. I could organize a dinner on Capitol Hill if you'll agree to speak and outline the needs."*

Broder quickly agreed to speak and to help arrange the event.

Over the next few weeks, Milken and Holden visited a number of medical research institutions and attended more medical meetings. At the annual meeting of the 15,000-member American Urological Association in San Antonio, they ran into Don Coffey again. Milken said he'd like to come see Coffey at Johns Hopkins. Coffey was typically self-effacing. *"Oh, I'm just a rat doctor, a Ph.D. I don't treat people. But if you'd like to see what we do in the lab, y'all come on up to Baltimore and we'll show you around."*

Milken didn't miss a beat. *"How's Tuesday morning?"*

Before long, Coffey was escorting Milken through his impressive laboratories at The Johns Hopkins Hospital and explaining his work on the role of the nuclear matrix in deoxyribonucleic acid (DNA) replication and hormone action. Milken asked Coffey about the growing impact of information technology on this work and soon they were deep into discussion of loop domains of DNA and other biological phenomena. No shrinking violet himself, Coffey was bowled over by Milken's energy. *"My colleagues are very accomplished people,"* notes Coffey. *"Most of them work on high octane. But when I met Mike Milken, I thought this guy works on jet fuel."*

Eventually, Skip Holden pulled Milken away with the suggestion that he should meet some of Coffey's protégés at the medical school. Milken questioned everyone he met about their work, their financial needs, the state of prostate cancer research, the role of the NCI and a head-spinning list of other topics. But first, he always wanted to know about their families, which he considered an important support network for researchers. Milken has drawn strength from his own family – his wife of 35 years and their three children.

One of the doctors he met at Hopkins was Jonathan Simons, M.D., who remembers it well:

> *"My wife, who is a Harvard-educated economist, tried to give me a small, but nonetheless trenchant explanation of how Mike had changed everything in terms of raising capital for new companies. My first impression was that this man was also going to change prostate cancer for the better."*

Heading north from Baltimore with Holden for their next meetings at New York's Memorial Sloan-Kettering Cancer Center, Milken mused out loud, "We may have to create something that doesn't exist."

"You mean a new organization?"

Milken's reply of "Maybe" was muffled as he buried his head in a newspaper.

"We can't just write checks"

A few days later, after visiting medical schools at Harvard and other East Coast universities, Milken and Holden were headed back to Los Angeles. "I remember the moment the Prostate Cancer Foundation was conceived," says Holden. "We were sitting on the plane and Mike suddenly blurted out, 'We can't just write checks.' By the time we landed, we had sketched out the plan for a new organization."

One fact was paramount in Milken's thinking: whatever had been done in the past hadn't worked. This new organization would have to break the mold. Holden explained that researchers were often spending 30 percent (and in some cases as much as 50 percent) of their time writing long and complex grant applications that met the NCI's exacting requirements – they were often hundreds of pages. Then it took a year to get approval; and another year to get the money. By that time, the grant applicant had often developed his work to the point where it was moving in a new direction. But under NCI rules, the research had to be exactly as specified in the original application, even if it had become less relevant.

Another problem was competition among institutions. Researchers too often saw medical research as a zero-sum game. There was just so much money to go around and if Johns Hopkins won a grant in a particular area of study, that meant that Sloan-Kettering and other centers were out of luck. This didn't exactly encourage collaboration across institutional boundaries.

Milken listened to all the problems, thought for a few minutes, and then scribbled down several requirements for the new organization:

- Identify the most promising research not being funded by the National Cancer Institute;
- Recruit the best scientists and physicians to energize the field;
- Limit awards applications to five pages;

- Make decisions on applications within 60 days and fund them in no more than 90 days;
- Require awardees to share the results of their work with other institutions;
- Help build *centers of excellence* at the nation's leading academic cancer centers and link them digitally;
- Get for-profit companies involved in collaboration with academic institutions and government agencies;
- Act with a sense of urgency;
- Build public awareness through advocacy programs.

There were other things to do – raising funds from the public, educating members of Congress, building coalitions – but the first priority was to jump-start new research. To that end, the Milken Family Foundation (MFF) made a $25-million commitment over five years to get the Prostate Cancer Foundation underway. (The MFF would later make a second $25-million commitment for another five years.) Although this was only a fraction of the hundreds of millions of dollars the MFF had given to education and medical research in previous years, it seemed revolutionary to prostate cancer researchers starved for government funding.

Smell the Flowers, But Hurry!

Much as Milken wanted to be directly involved in the operations of the Prostate Cancer Foundation, there was the little matter of staying alive. He had to pursue an aggressive course of treatment. He also knew from decades of working in philanthropy that it takes a professional staff and an active, involved board of directors to make any charitable organization effective.

Milken's brother-in-law, Allen Flans, a retired endodontist with business experience, understood the healthcare field and was eager to lend a hand in getting the new foundation up and running. Installed as the PCF's initial executive director, Flans quickly hired a professional staff. Skip Holden agreed to be the medical director and establish a research strategy. Milken himself recruited a board of directors comprising a mix of distinguished physicians, philanthropists and colleagues from his previous business endeavors, as well as sports, political and entertainment figures. Some of the board members had the additional qualification of being prostate cancer survivors.

With a structure in place and initial funding assured for the Prostate Cancer Foundation, Milken could focus on his own treatment. Surgery to remove his prostate was not an option since his cancer had already escaped the prostate and spread to his lymph nodes. Bad as his prognosis sounded, it would be worse if cancer cells had invaded his bones. A bone-marrow test was conducted at M.D. Anderson Cancer Center in Houston by Christopher Logothetis, M.D., who would later become chairman of the center's department of genitourinary medical oncology. At last there was some encouraging news: Milken's bones were clear.

In addition to M.D. Anderson, Milken consulted doctors and had further tests at Johns Hopkins, the University of Virginia and Memorial Sloan-Kettering Cancer Center in New York, where another lymph-node biopsy was conducted under general anesthesia. The Sloan-Kettering doctors injected cancer cells from Milken's lymph nodes into a mouse in an attempt to create a cell line of his tumor that could act as a target for further therapies. It was a long shot and it didn't work.

Skip Holden put Milken on androgen-deprivation therapy, a medical strategy that deprives the cancer cells of the male hormones they need to proliferate. It would take several months of this therapy, which involved taking two pills three times every day and getting a monthly injection, to bring his PSA count down to a level that indicated the cancer cells were at least temporarily weakened.

The next step was eight weeks of three-dimensional conformal external-beam radiation of his prostate and pelvic lymph nodes. This therapy uses computers to create a 3D picture that allows multiple radiation beams to conform precisely to the contour of the treatment area. The goal was to eradicate any residual cancer that wasn't eliminated by the hormonal treatment. Milken understood that if these two therapies failed, no other consistently effective treatment options were available to him.

Fortunately for Milken, his response to the treatments was "dramatic," as described by *Time* magazine:

> "His PSA level dropped from 24 to 15, then to 10, 5 and 3. When he began supplementary radiation therapy [in the fall of 1993], it stood at zero. The computer scans were also encouraging; they showed that his swollen lymph nodes had shrunk back to normal size. Milken's cancer was, and still is, in remission. But Milken is realistic. He knows that in men who have undergone hormone therapy, the cancer cells eventually learn to thrive. While Milken has reacted unusually well to treatment, he is all too aware that he has not been cured. 'We just don't know how long before it comes back,' he says."

Try to relax

Between the time he started hormone therapy in the spring and radiation late that fall, Milken made trips to several medical centers and visited biotechnology and pharmaceutical companies with his wife, Lori. Meeting with the CEOs of several companies, including Gordon Binder at Amgen and William Haseltine at Human Genome Sciences, Milken argued that more of their resources should be directed to fighting cancer:

> "It was déjà vu for me. Two decades earlier, I had traveled the country talking about the need to open up access to capital through the use of new financial technologies including non-investment-grade debt instruments. Now I was on the road again, telling executives that medical costs are the largest and fastest-growing sector of our economy; that our population is aging; that cancer is a major problem that will only get worse; and that they should be doing more research in that area."

Milken also made changes in his lifestyle. Able to function in top form with only a few hours sleep a night, he had always maintained a pace that would have exhausted most people. But faced with a terminal prognosis, he said he was going to try to slow down and relax more. It occurred to him that every one of his relatives who had been stricken with cancer had passively followed the traditional regimens of Western medicine. And every one of them was dead. What could he do that they had not?

To begin, he swore off his lifetime habit of eating high-fat foods like meat and dairy products. After months of surviving on steamed vegetables and fresh fruit, he began to have dreams about hot dogs, lasagna and chocolate pudding. But with his life on the line, he stuck to his drab diet. A few years later, he figured out how to enjoy his favorite foods without compromising his health (see Chapter 11).

He then studied and embraced several alternative concepts including meditation, sesame-oil massages, aromatherapy and yoga. Without rejecting traditional Western medicine, he figured that these non-traditional methods were at worst harmless and might even help. Certain aromas, including the salt air of the seashore and the pine needles of a mountain forest, were found to raise his T-cells, a measure of his immune system's strength.

During that spring of 1993, Milken read Norman Cousins' inspiring book *Anatomy of an Illness*. He talked at length with Hamilton Jordan, the White House Chief of Staff in the Carter Administration, who had already dealt with two types of cancer and who had strong views about how a patient should take charge of his treatment. (Two years later, they would reverse roles when Jordan would be diagnosed with a third cancer – in his prostate – and Milken advised him on the leading surgeons.)

Mike and Lori spent a week at the Maharishi Center in the Berkshire Mountains of western Massachusetts with Indian Ayurvedic medical practitioners to learn more about alternative therapies. He consulted with Dr. Deepak Chopra, the author and leader of the Chopra Center, which was then also located in Massachusetts. Later, he moved an Ayurvedic physician into his house for several months to supervise alternative therapies in conjunction with traditional Western medical treatments.

> *"For me, this began a period of embracing Eastern medicine,"* Milken recalls. *"I went to Russia in the summer of 1994 and met with a healer. The next year I was in China to interact with 'chi' doctors. I felt it was important to connect the mind with the body. I got my family involved and met with people like Dr. Chopra. I spent a lot of time meditating and going to the beach. I put a water fountain outside the windows in my library so that I could hear the sound of water as I read."*

There was even time to smell the flowers, literally, as Mike and Lori took a vacation that included visits to gardens in Holland and other countries. Eleven years later, Milken's PSA count is zero, he appears healthy, and he continues to work 15 hours a day. Asked which therapies he credits for his good health, he candidly

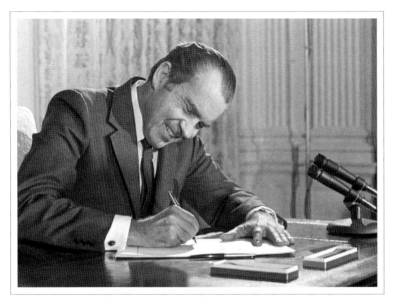

President Richard Nixon signed the National Cancer Act in 1971, and declared War on Cancer.

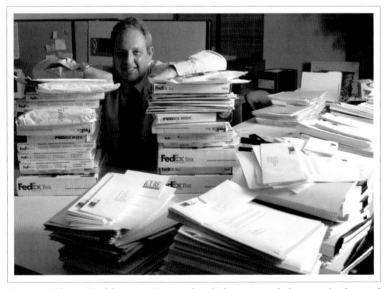

Stuart "Skip" Holden, M.D., medical director of the newly formed Prostate Cancer Foundation, with some of the organization's first award applications.

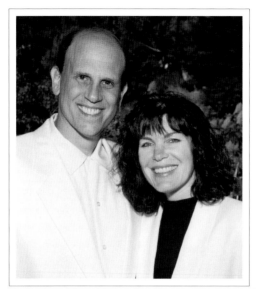

Mike and Lori Milken soon after Mike was diagnosed with advanced prostate cancer in 1993. Twenty-one years earlier, Lori's mother had been diagnosed with breast cancer, the event that sparked Mike's three decades of involvement in medical research and philanthropy.

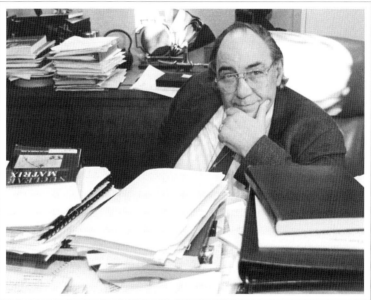

One of the first researchers Mike Milken met after his prostate cancer diagnosis was Donald Coffey, Ph.D., considered to be *the father of prostate cancer research in America.*" A professor at Johns Hopkins School of Medicine, Coffey is former president of the American Association for Cancer Research.

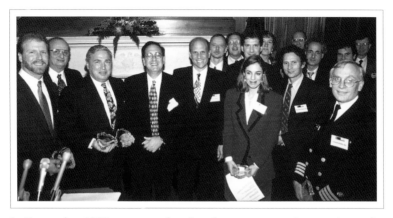

In September 1993 – six months after the organization's inception – the Prostate Cancer Foundation announced that 30 competitive research awards totaling $4.5 million would go to researchers at 26 institutions in 14 states. In November, the winners convened in the Mansfield Room of the U.S. Capitol at the PCF's first Call-to-Action Dinner to receive their awards.

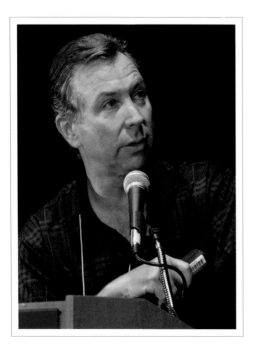

One of the first PCF-supported researchers was 1993 Research Award winner Neil Bander, M.D., at the New York Hospital, Cornell Medical Center. Bander produced monoclonal antibodies to PSMA (prostate-specific membrane antigen), which through continuing research has led to clinical trials exploring potential effects on prostate cancer cells.

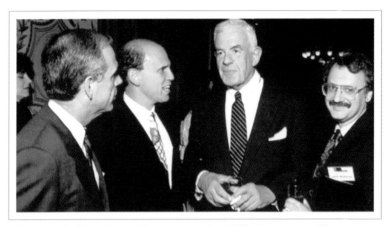

The 1993 Call-to-Action Dinner was the PCF's first major effort to raise awareness of prostate cancer in Washington. Left to right: California Congressman Tony Coehlo; PCF Chairman Mike Milken; Speaker of the House Tom Foley; and then-director of the National Cancer Institute, Sam Broder, M.D.

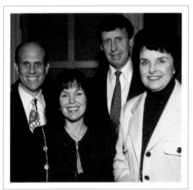

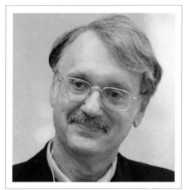

U.S. Senator Dianne Feinstein (right), who lost her former husband to cancer and has been a leading supporter of cancer research, was one of many U.S. senators and representatives to attend the PCF's 1993 Call-to-Action Dinner. Above, Feinstein with Mike and Lori Milken and her husband, Richard Blum.

Sam Broder, M.D., helped the Milken Family Foundation establish its Cancer Research Awards in the 1980s. He later became Director of the National Cancer Institute. Dr. Broder is now Chief Medical Officer of Celera Genomics, which completed the first draft sequence of the human genome.

The Milken Family Foundation, established in 1982 to formalize the previous philanthropy of Michael and Lowell Milken, has supported a broad range of medical research. One of its programs, the Cancer Research Awards, provided individual grants ranging up to $250,000. Some winners are shown below.

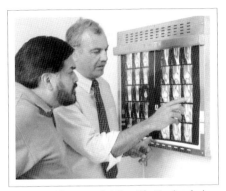

Dennis Slamon, M.D., Ph.D. (right), a researcher at the University of California, Los Angeles, discovered Herceptin, a revolutionary breakthrough treatment for one type of breast cancer.

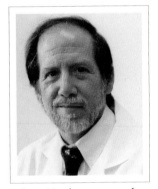

Johns Hopkins researcher, Bert Vogelstein, M.D., pioneered work on the crucial p53 gene whose mutant form is believed to be linked to more than half of human cancers.

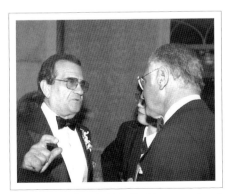

Ernst Wynder, M.D, (left) is credited with co-authoring the first study definitively linking lung cancer and smoking in the 1950s. He received a Milken Family Foundation Cancer Research award in 1990.

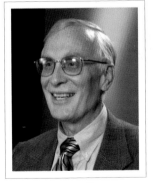

Charles 'Snuffy' Myers, M.D., then Chief of the Clinical Pharmacology branch of the NCI, today heads the American Institute for Diseases of the Prostate.

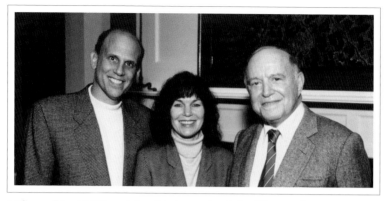

Mike and Lori Milken joined industrialist John Kluge at his 14,000-acre Charlottesville farm, where Kluge hosted a strategy session the day after the 1993 Call-to-Action Dinner. More than 40 leading prostate cancer researchers, industry and business leaders, prostate cancer survivors and government officials participated.

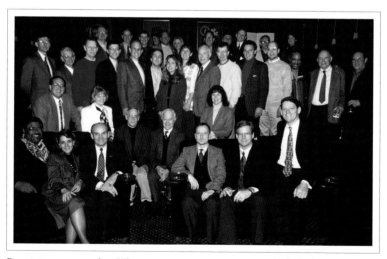

Participants at the Kluge strategy session concluded that medical research for all diseases was significantly underfunded, that the drug-approval process should be accelerated, that new incentives were needed to attract young investigators to research careers, and that researchers at different institutions and in different disciplines needed to break out of their "silo mentality" and collaborate more. As researchers expressed their frustration at the lack of funding, Mike Milken rose to say, "Your job is to do the science. My job is to get the money."

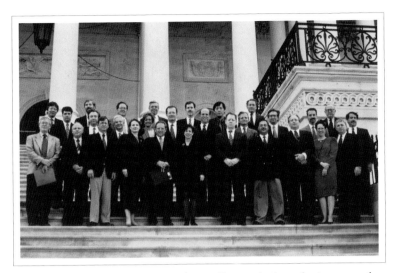

The 1994 Prostate Cancer Foundation Research Award winners gather on the U.S. Capitol steps. Forty-six competitive research awards totaling $4.8 million were announced.

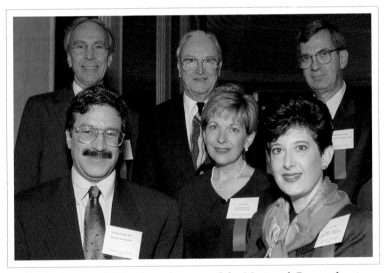

Richard Klausner, M.D., then-director of the National Cancer Institute (front left) was joined at the National Cancer Summit by former NCI directors (back row) Arthur Upton, M.D., Carl Baker, M.D., and Vincent DeVita Jr., M.D.; and Ellen Stovall, executive director of the National Coalition for Cancer Survivorship and Amy Langer of the Breast Cancer Alliance (right).

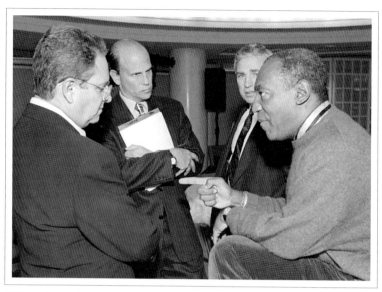

Bill Cosby at the 1993 Call-to-Action Dinner with PCF Medical Director Skip Holden, M.D., Mike Milken and Andrew von Eschenbach, M.D., then a leading urologist at the M.D. Anderson Cancer Center. Von Eschenbach would later be appointed Director of the National Cancer Institute. Cosby is one of hundreds of celebrities who have donated time and talent for the PCF cause.

Quincy Jones speaks at one of the Prostate Cancer Foundation's first fund-raisers, held at the Pickfair estate, once the home of Douglas Fairbanks Jr. and Mary Pickford, in Los Angeles.

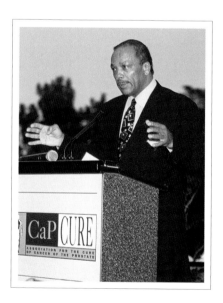

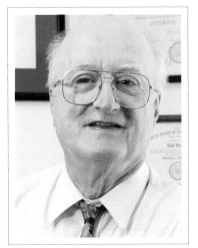

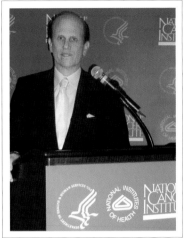

The PCF sponsored a 1995 Working Meeting on Standards to encourage faster release of oncology drugs. Emil Frei, M.D., Physician-in-Chief Emeritus at Dana-Farber Cancer Institute, summed up the meeting: *"We have formed the basis of a major change in clinical trials and a major improvement and acceleration of progress in cancer treatment."*

In January 2004, Prostate Cancer Foundation Chairman Mike Milken addressed a crucial National Cancer Institute roundtable convened to refine America's national strategy for reducing the burden of cancer. The roundtable developed what the NCI's Director called *"a wealth of substantive solutions."*

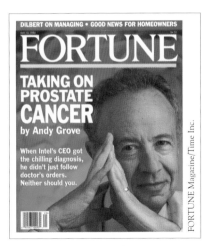

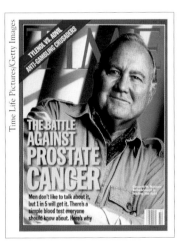

PCF efforts to increase public awareness of prostate cancer got a boost in early 1996 when two prominent prostate cancer survivors were featured on the covers of national magazines.

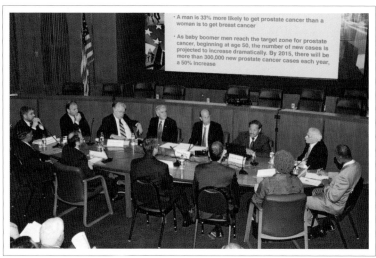

PCF President and CEO Leslie Michelson (second from right, top row) presents epidemiological data about prostate cancer to a roundtable meeting called by the Majority Leader of the New York State Senate, Joseph Bruno (fourth from left, top row). The meeting helped develop support for a bill that would allow New York taxpayers to check a box on their state tax returns directing that their refunds be sent to a non-profit organization funding prostate cancer research. The State Senate later passed the bill 60-0.

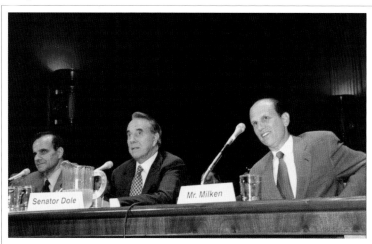

New York Yankees Manager Joe Torre, former Senator Bob Dole and Mike Milken testified before the U.S. Senate Subcommittee on Labor, Health & Human Services and Education Appropriations in 1999 to urge the government to fund more cancer research.

admits he doesn't know. "I was willing to try anything that had the potential to work. Today, I take my prescribed medications, eat a very healthy diet, exercise, and try to keep everything in perspective. I also speak to cancer patients every day. When I can be helpful, it's as rewarding for me as it is for them."

Up and running

Throughout his treatment, Milken was staying close to developments at the Prostate Cancer Foundation and meeting regularly with leaders in the field of prostate cancer. He soon concluded that some of the leading medical centers in the country were not really centers of excellence in prostate cancer. He cites Harvard as an example:

> "Their grouping of research institutes, the medical school and several hospitals is one of the elite medical complexes in the world. I met with several Harvard medical executives in 1993, including their director of development, and told them they didn't have a competitive program for the most common cancer in American men. This should have been a concern to them if only because prostate cancer was going to affect their wealthy donors, who would then turn to other institutions for treatment. They doubted that this was a big problem, so I challenged them to conduct a survey of their donors asking them to rank their medical concerns. To their surprise, the survey showed that the number-one concern was back pain. And what was number two? Prostate cancer!"

Researchers at Harvard had submitted almost no applications for PCF competitive research grants in 1993. Following the survey of their donors, applications picked up and in 1995 Harvard sent the PCF more applications than any other institution.

Milken concluded that a key PCF strategy would be to focus on building centers of excellence that would be leaders in pursuing the most advanced science. He believed it was disruptive and counterproductive for institutions to keep bidding against each other for the limited pool of top talent. The way to create value and accelerate science, he said, was to recruit more of the best and brightest graduates into medical research careers. That way, the leading centers could maintain continuity in their research programs. Milken drove home this theme during the PCF's early years with talks at the Dana Farber Cancer Center, UCLA, M.D. Anderson Cancer Center, the University of Virginia, and Johns Hopkins University among others. He offered to help them raise money and bond with their donors. Perhaps the most striking example of this focus on "human capital" is the University of California at San Francisco, whose development as a center of excellence in prostate cancer is described in Chapter 8.

Milken knew that medical scientists wouldn't pursue careers in prostate cancer if money wasn't available for research. He discussed this with Patrick Walsh, M.D., urologist-in-chief at Johns Hopkins, who pioneered nerve-sparing prostate surgery. Walsh is best known to laymen as the author of *Dr. Patrick Walsh's Guide to Surviving Prostate Cancer.*

> *"Mike outlined the strategy to turn things around,"* says Walsh. *"It was really very simple: he said there are too few people applying for grants in prostate cancer, and when the grants are received, there are too few people qualified to review them. And so there are too few grants being funded and there are too few investigators in the field. He said if we make money available, there will be more investigators. And that's exactly what happened."*

Within weeks of its establishment in the spring of 1993, the PCF had initiated a competitive research awards program and organized a review board of leading scientists and physicians to screen the applications. By July, they had received 86 applications and, true to their word, they moved quickly. In less than a month, the PCF announced the first 30 awards totaling $4.5 million to researchers at 26 institutions in 14 states. Some grants went to experienced scientists with long, distinguished resumes – more than one would go to a Nobel laureate. But Dr. Walsh remembers in particular the impact on more-recent graduates:

"There were a lot of really talented young investigators who could have been working in any field. They weren't working in prostate cancer because there wasn't any money. All of a sudden, there was opportunity with a relatively simple, rapid-review process to apply for funding. And so young investigators without a track record, who would have had a great deal of difficulty receiving funding from the government, were able to get funding to try out pilot projects. And these individuals solidified their careers in this field because of the opportunity for funding, and then, once the government caught on, were able to get continued funding."

One of the first recipients of a Prostate Cancer Foundation grant was Jonathan Simons, the young research physician Milken had met at Johns Hopkins a few months earlier. Simons, a former Rhodes Scholar who now heads the Winship Cancer Institute at Emory University in Atlanta, credits early PCF awards with a "fulcrum effect" – a lever that lifted the world of prostate cancer research:

"In 2003, we competed with 13 other institutions and got a $10-million Defense Department grant for prostate cancer research here at Emory, the largest three-year grant in the history of prostate cancer research. Every single person on this grant has received PCF funding in the past – every single one. If you took all the PCF awards starting back in 1993 and looked downstream at all the government funding that grew from it – add it all up and I bet the return on investment would be pretty amazing."

In choosing which applications should be funded, the PCF review board – a group of highly respected physicians and scientists – wanted to encourage novel approaches. They took a portfolio approach identifying a number of experimental therapeutic strategies that they felt were most promising:

- Anti-angiogenesis (cutting blood supply to tumors);
- Vaccines and gene therapy;
- Nutritional studies;
- Studies of apoptosis (the process of cell death);
- Therapies targeting the androgen receptor.

As Holden put it, *"We said, in effect, send us the novel ideas you haven't sent to the National Cancer Institute. We wanted to help the NCI by doing preliminary proofs of ideas. We never claimed to be like the NCI. We had a different mission and a greater sense of urgency."*

The grant process was as revolutionary as it was simple: send five pages, tell us what you're going to do and why it's important; we'll reply within 60 days and, if we approve, send the money within 90 days. This encouraged the best and the brightest to send their ideas. A number of these researchers said later that they would not have bothered with the National Cancer Institute's laborious and time-consuming application process for certain projects, especially since the probability of funding was small. But the PCF's streamlined process and openness to new ideas stimulated their creativity and ultimately accelerated the science.

Raising the Profile

*F*rom day one, everyone involved with the Prostate Cancer Foundation has understood the importance of attracting leading researchers and supporting the early development of their innovative ideas. Some of these ideas will fall by the wayside; but many others will be shown to have validity, which will qualify them for much larger funding by private industry and government agencies. This is the concept of *venture funding*. A relatively modest award of a few hundred thousand dollars from the PCF can be leveraged many times over when it is used to develop an idea to the point where it attracts millions of government dollars.

Back in 1993, however, the portion of the Federal budget allocated to all medical research was small – about a third of what it is today – and the $2 billion spent on all cancer research was less than the 1993 cost – $3.5 billion – of a single aircraft carrier. Funds for prostate cancer were almost nonexistent. Today, federal, state and local government agencies invest close to $6 billion in cancer research, of which close to $500 million a year goes to prostate cancer research. That's almost 20 times the 1993 level for prostate cancer. The Prostate Cancer Foundation has helped raise awareness of the fact that investments in medical research return enormous dividends to society.

The first awareness-raising event was a November 1993 "Call-to-Action" dinner, hosted by Milken and PCF Executive Director Allen Flans in the ornate Mansfield Room of the U.S. Capitol. The PCF wanted to bring together the winners of its first competitive research awards with several members of Congress and federal agency executives to showcase the importance of increasing federal research spending. It also wanted to provide a high level of recognition and respect for under-appreciated scientists.

This focus on recognition was nothing new for the Milkens. Since the mid-1980s, the Milken Family Foundation, headed by Lowell Milken, had been recognizing hundreds of outstanding teachers across the country by bringing them to a gala awards ceremony in Los Angeles and presenting each of them with an unrestricted $25,000 prize. The idea was that there are Academy Awards for actors, MVP awards for athletes, Grammys for musicians, Pulitzer Prizes for journalists and so on; so why not a national award for the best teachers, the very people who educate all the other award winners? The Foundation carried this concept into the field of medicine, where awards to young investigators had recognized outstanding researchers for several years.

> *"I'll never forget that evening back in 1993,"* recalls Andrew von Eschenbach. *"Walking up the Capitol steps and seeing that beautiful light on the dome and the gleaming white marble, I was awestruck. I couldn't believe that this kid from South Philly was walking into the Capitol of the United States of America and actually going to have dinner there. I only wish that my Dad, who died from prostate cancer, could have been there with me. But in a way he was."*

Among the 100 invited guests who attended were U.S. Senators William Cohen, Bob Dole, Dianne Feinstein, Jake Garn, John Glenn, Richard Shelby and Ted Stevens; Speaker of the House Tom Foley; former House Democratic whip Tony Coelho; columnist Robert Novak; former professional football star Rosey Grier; entertainer and record producer Quincy Jones; National Cancer Institute Director Sam Broder; Dr. Emil Frei, a legend in cancer research and Physician-in-Chief Emeritus of the Dana Farber Cancer Institute; and more than 50 other researchers from major medical centers across the country.

It was an emotional evening for everyone involved. But it was also a powerful statement that medical research should receive more attention – that despite the dashing of false hopes that had often been raised about a potential cancer cure, here was a group of incredibly impressive researchers who believed strongly in the value of the work they were doing. The members of Congress in the Mansfield Room that night were clearly moved by what they heard. They sensed that changes were coming in the field of cancer research and they renewed their commitment to advocate increased federal funding.

No more filing cabinets

Following a warm introduction by Quincy Jones, Milken told the audience how irrational it seemed to spend $100 billion annually in the U.S. on cancer and dedicate only about $2 billion to finding a cure. The rest was for patient care. *"Is there an example anywhere in private industry,"* he asked, *"where a company would spend 50 times as much to deal with the consequences of a problem as it would to solve the problem? It just doesn't make sense."*

Milken also commented on proposed legislation that threatened to increase the regulatory burden on the healthcare industry, a threat that could force companies to reduce their drug research budgets. Then he addressed the bureaucratic process that slows the search for medical solutions. *"Many people have submitted grant applications [to the government] that are bulky enough to fill entire filing cabinets. How long and how much energy does it take to produce a filing cabinet full of paper to ask for a grant? By the time you've filled that cabinet, you're worn out."* He noted pointedly that the Prostate Cancer Foundation required only a five-page application.

NCI Director Broder spoke of the need for greater commitment to research:

> *"This is not an intellectual game; it's a matter of life and death. We must have no illusions about how difficult our task is ... It is exceedingly important for us to recall the unity of all cancer research and to look for innovative ways to find new discoveries from unexpected opportunities. There is a profound interrela-*

tionship between certain forms of cancer. It is impossible to make progress against one cancer without making progress against all."

The following day, an article in the *Washington Post* reported that *"Broder told the audience the battle against prostate cancer may be won because of Milken's leadership."*

They gasped

From Washington, the 1993 PCF award winners traveled 100 miles southwest for a strategy session at the 14,000-acre Charlottesville, Virginia farm of John Kluge. Almost a decade earlier, Milken had arranged what was then the largest public financing in the history of financial markets for Metromedia, the company Kluge had founded. As a prostate cancer survivor, Kluge was happy to host an event that could advance the cause of cancer research.

At Milken's invitation, industry leaders like Carl Lindner and Nelson Peltz (with his wife, Claudia) had attended the Washington dinner and then joined the researchers in Charlottesville. As with the Mansfield Room dinner, Milken wanted all the award winners to be treated in a way that showed recognition and appreciation for their outstanding work.

One of the hosts for the meeting was Jay Gillenwater, M.D., editor of the Journal of Urology, professor of urology at the University of Virginia Health Science Center, and an expert in the use of radioactive seed implantation to treat prostate cancer. As president of the American Urological Association, Gillenwater had met Milken earlier in the year at the AUA's annual meeting in San Antonio. Among other participants in Charlottesville were David McCloud, M.D., J.D., chief of urologic oncology at Walter Reed Army Medical Center; and Donna Peehl, Ph.D., associate professor of urology at Stanford University Medical School, who is widely known for developing the methodology for the culture of prostate cells.

The meeting was designed as a roundtable discussion that would debate the direction and funding of prostate cancer research and map out the most important needs going forward. Everyone agreed that medical research for all diseases was significantly underfunded, that the drug-approval process should be accelerated, that new incentives were needed to attract young investigators to research careers, and that researchers at different institutions and in different disciplines needed to break out of their "silo mentality" and collaborate more.

Several of the doctors talked about the frustration and distraction of constantly searching for the next grant to continue their research. Finally, Milken stood up and said something that none of the medical scientists in the room had ever heard before:

"Your job is to do the science. My job is to get the money."

There was a collective gasp. No one could believe what they'd just heard. Milken's point was that these brilliant doctors were wasting at least a third of their time raising money. If they could be freed of that burden, the science would move faster. The way he saw it, the PCF should be able to increase their productivity as much as 50 percent by giving them back a third of their time to add to the two-thirds they spent doing research.

Over the next decade, the Prostate Cancer Foundation would make good on that pledge in several ways. It raised enough money on its own to fund more than 1,100 medical research projects. But it participated with other organizations in advocacy campaigns that helped to more than triple the budget of the National Institutes of Health to $27 billion by 2003; it pushed for increased spending on prostate cancer by both the National Cancer Institute and state health agencies nationwide; it backed the creation of the Prostate Cancer Research Program in the Department of Defense; and it encouraged dozens of new investments by pharmaceutical and biotechnology companies in prostate cancer and other medical therapies.

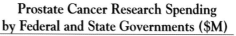

**Prostate Cancer Research Spending
by Federal and State Governments ($M)**

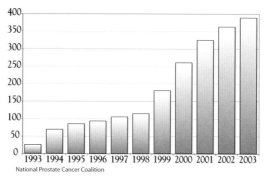

National Prostate Cancer Coalition

People are sometimes surprised to hear that the Department of Defense (DoD) has a large prostate-cancer research program. Military recruitment advertising shows healthy young men and women in uniform. But as military men age, a significant number of them are diagnosed with prostate cancer and many of them die. Before the mid-1990s, the Defense Department had no prostate cancer research programs. It occurred to Milken that the DoD, with its huge budget, could emulate the biomedical initiatives of the National Aeronautics and Space Administration, which studied such phenomena as the effects of space flight on the human body. Early in 1994, he asked a longtime friend, California Congressman Tom Lantos, to introduce him to NASA Administrator Dan Goldin. As Goldin outlined NASA's medical research, Milken wondered if similar programs could be started in the Defense Department to work on cancer.

Over the next two years, PCF representatives met with more than 100 members of Congress to encourage support for increased cancer research. Some of this work was coordinated with advocates for breast cancer research, who were leading an effort for funding by the DoD. This led to multiple Congressional resolutions urging increased appropriations and better coordination of government programs. Meanwhile, PCF board member and Intel Chairman Andy Grove became an effective advocate for a Department of Defense research program.

Finally, in late 1996, Congress approved a Defense Department program of prostate cancer research – a $45-million appropriation for 1997. Grove and PCF executives then met with Dr. Richard Klausner, the director of the National Cancer Institute, to discuss how the NCI's programs could most effectively coordinate with those at the DoD's Prostate Cancer Research Program (PCRP). By 2003, the PCRP had provided a total of $395 million for more than 800 peer-reviewed projects. Holden helped determine the program's goals as a member of its integration panel.

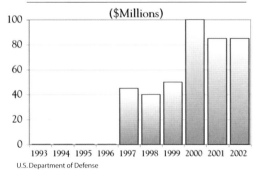

Defense Department Spending on the Prostate Cancer Research Program

($Millions)

U.S. Department of Defense

The PCRP's largest single grant of $10 million went to two researchers whose work had been supported by the Prostate Cancer Foundation for many years: Jonathan Simons, M.D. (see Chapter 4) and Leland Chung, Ph.D., at Emory University. The manager of the PCRP, Leo Giambarresi, Ph.D., of the U.S. Army says, *"There would not have been a DoD prostate cancer research program without the efforts of the Prostate Cancer Foundation and Mike Milken. He has done more to increase funding and awareness of prostate cancer than anyone."*

One of the PCF's original strategies was to help build centers of excellence at the top medical institutions and urge the NCI to establish more federal funding for so-called SPORE grants for all cancers.

SPOREs – Specialized Programs of Research Excellence – are NCI-funded grants that support innovative, multidisciplinary translational research approaches that potentially may have an immediate impact on improving cancer care and prevention. They are a clear affirmation that a medical center has "made it" to the elite circle of the world's best. The result of the campaign for more SPOREs has been profound. In 1992, there were only two such prostate cancer programs: at the Baylor College of Medicine and at Johns Hopkins University. By 2004, there were 11 prostate cancer SPOREs and the number of SPORE grants for all cancers had increased from 9 to 62 with prostate cancer having the largest number.

Number of SPORE Grants

	1992-3	1995-6	1999	2000	2001	2002	2003	2004
Breast	4	6	6	9	9	9	9	10
Prostate	**2**	**3**	**3**	**4**	**8**	**11**	**11**	**11**
Lung	2	3	3	3	6	6	7	7
Gastro-Intestinal	1	2	2	2	2	4	4	6
Ovary	-	-	4	4	4	4	4	5
GU	-	-	-	-	1	1	2	2
Skin	-	-	-	-	1	2	2	3
Brain	-	-	-	-	-	2	2	4
H&N	-	-	-	-	-	3	3	4
Lymphoma	-	-	-	-	-	2	2	3
GYN	-	-	-	-	-	-	2	2
Leukemia	-	-	-	-	-	-	1	1
Myeloma	-	-	-	-	-	-	1	1
Pancreas	-	-	-	-	-	-	3	3
Total Programs	9	14	18	22	31	44	54	62
Total Budgets ($M)	$20	$30	$39	$48	$68	$112	$121	$140

Source: National Cancer Institute

Meanwhile, the PCF had been continuing its efforts to raise awareness in Washington. At its second "Call-to-Action" dinner in 1994, the Foundation announced another $4.8 million in funding for 46 new research projects to an audience that included Senators John Chafee, William Cohen, Bob Dole, Orrin Hatch, Richard Shelby and Ted Stevens, as well as Representatives Julian Dixon, Pete Stark, Maxine Waters and Ron Wyden. A year later, Bill Cosby served as master of ceremonies for the 1995 dinner and announced that funding had grown to $10.2 million for 62 competitive awards including, for the first time, grants to medical institutions outside the U.S.

Internationalization of the research effort has always been a key theme at the PCF. Over the years since the 1995 awards, researchers in ten nations other than the United States have been funded: Australia, Austria, Canada, Finland, Germany, Israel, the Netherlands, Scotland, Sweden and Switzerland. The case of Israel shows how these investments have been made strategically to stimulate further investment in particular areas.

Israel has the world's highest percentage of citizens with university and advanced degrees. After the fall of the Soviet Union, a large number of Russian scientists moved to Israel, further expanding its human capital of highly educated people. The PCF saw an opportunity to focus these scientists on prostate cancer. Through the generosity of a PCF board member, it was possible to create a critical mass of funding that eventually would lead to collaborative efforts in 11 Israeli academic centers:

- Assaf Harofe Medical Center
- Bar-Ilan University
- Ben-Gurion University of the Negev
- Hadassah University
- Hebrew University
- Rabin Medical Center
- Sheba Medical Center
- Technion, Israel Institute of Technology
- Tel-Aviv University
- Volcani Center
- Weizmann Institute of Science

"In Israel, there was practically nothing earmarked for prostate cancer several years ago," says Yosef Yarden, Ph.D., a PCF award-winning researcher at the Weizmann Institute of Science. *"The PCF changed the situation dramatically in this country. Now, the European community is putting large sums into prostate cancer research, and there's a major effort to*

assemble clinical centers under the same umbrella. In Israel, the effect is without precedent. Ten years ago there was maybe 10 percent of what we have now. PCF grants have attracted large numbers of people to the field. Let's call it catalytic money – money invested in a smart way. Once researchers are in the field, they manage to raise money from other sources."

Seeking better standards

By 1995, the PCF had become a recognized force in the medical community, not only for its ability to raise funds, but also for its strategy of fostering collaboration among researchers at diverse institutions. But the clinical community of practicing physicians still felt that too many patients were dying from cancer without being given an opportunity to try experimental drugs that had shown effectiveness in early testing.

The Food and Drug Administration protects patients by preventing marketing of drugs for general use until they have gone through several phases of carefully controlled testing to determine safety and dosage (Phase I); evaluate effectiveness and look for side effects (Phase II); and confirm effectiveness ("efficacy") while identifying any adverse reactions from long-term use (Phase III). The problem is that with prostate-cancer drugs it takes a very long time – usually many years – to prove efficacy in Phase III because prostate cancer often progresses slowly. As a result, a new drug shown to be safe in Phase I and effective in Phase II might be unavailable to most patients – even those near death – until years later when the FDA has acted on Phase III data. This delay frustrated cancer doctors, their patients and the patients' families. An editorial in the *Canadian Medical Association Journal*, under the headline "Patience is a luxury of the well," reported Milken's view:

"[He] has argued that the medical and scientific establishment in North America should approach cancer research with more urgency. Milken is typical of patients with prostate cancer. They want results. They don't want progress to be held up by inefficient bureaucracies or interdisciplinary politicking.

Although they recognize the need for proper scientific investigation of new treatments, they do not want such investigations to drag on interminably when it is clear to all involved that clinical benefits are available."

During the summer of 1995, Milken had met at Lake Tahoe with Colin Powell, the former chairman of the Joint Chiefs of Staff (and future Secretary of State) to urge him to assume the leadership of the cancer advocacy movement. As they discussed how the War on Cancer should proceed, Powell cited the philosophy of the commander on the ground in the 1991 Gulf War, General Norman Schwarzkopf: you never have all the information you need about an enemy, but you have to move forward with the best information and tools available. Milken saw a clear parallel in the use of experimental drugs to treat cancer – if we know a drug provides benefits, we shouldn't wait until we have perfect information before allowing its use for desperately ill patients.

The PCF addressed this issue later that summer by sponsoring a "Working Meeting on Standards" in Washington to encourage the more rapid release of oncology drugs. Some 50 representatives from academic institutions, the FDA, the NCI and advocacy communities attended.

"This effort was to determine if we could treat cancer drugs differently than we treat medicines for back pain, arthritis and other types of diseases that might have to go to Phase III clinical trials," says Milken. *"With some diseases, you can withhold treatment for a year and you're still OK. Not so with cancer – people are dying. If I've got a one- to two-year life expectancy, why can't I try a drug that has worked in Phase II? Our message to the FDA was that we should work as a team to accelerate cancer research."*

Among other recommendations, the conference proposed:

- Pre-clinical information requirements for Phase I trials should be reasonable, but not exhaustive;

- Phase I trials should be flexible, tailored to the therapeutic candidate, and encouraging toward new approaches that maximize potential benefits to patients;
- Phase I trials should not only assess toxicology issues, but also determine biological and therapeutic effects as a function of drug dosage and drug schedule;
- Third-party payers should reimburse the expenses of cancer patients enrolled in all phases of clinical trials involving new uses of approved drugs;
- Independent symposia to educate physicians about new uses of chemotherapeutic agents should be encouraged … and supported by pharmaceutical companies;
- Development time of Phase II and Phase III trials should be radically shortened and barriers to physician and patient participation should be removed;
- Surrogate markers [test results, such as those from a PSA test, that don't prove the absence or existence of a condition, but tend be highly correlated with it] may suffice for regulatory approval, with a requirement for additional studies on survival time.

Emil Frei, III, M.D., Physician-in-Chief Emeritus at the Dana-Farber Cancer Institute, in whose name the Milken Family Foundation had endowed a chair at Harvard a decade earlier, played a leadership role in the standards meeting. A few days later, he wrote:

> *"I believe that we have formed the basis of a major change in clinical trials and a major improvement and acceleration of progress in cancer treatment. The positive and enthusiastic thrust of the Prostate Cancer Foundation is quite in contrast to the pessimistic mood that pervades much of cancer research at the moment."*

There was encouraging agreement that the process of drug approvals could be improved. The meeting's recommendations were summarized in a white paper that the PCF and other organizations circulated to key decision makers in the Administration and on Capitol Hill. But it would take more to turn agreement into action.

United We Stand

*F*ollowing up on the momentum generated by the Working Meeting on Standards during the summer of 1995, the PCF immediately began planning a broader meeting – a Cancer Summit – to raise Washington's awareness that cancer will strike 100 million Americans and to show unity across several cancer organizations. The November 14th Summit was co-sponsored by the PCF, the National Coalition for Cancer Survivorship (NCCS), the National Alliance of Breast Cancer Organizations, former Surgeon General C. Everett Koop, U.S. Secretary of Education Richard Riley, and 44 spouses of U.S. Senators.

The Summit was quite a logistical accomplishment since the entire U.S. Government had virtually shut down that day in response to the failure of Congress to pass an omnibus appropriations bill. Of course, the press had a field day with that, showing empty office buildings and providing a forum for partisan bickering. Democrats blamed Republicans for holding up the people's business, and Republicans attacked Democrats for budget deficits. In the midst of this, Milken was scheduled to appear on NBC's *Today Show* in connection with the Cancer Summit.

Listening with an earpiece as he was waiting to be interviewed in a hotel hallway outside the Summit, Milken heard the previous *Today Show* guest, Speaker of the House Newt Gingrich, assail political opponents for "leaving future generations with the burden of a huge government debt." Moments later, Milken was on the air telling a national audience that we should indeed be concerned about what we leave to future generations. But he wasn't talking about budget deficits.

"My parents' generation fought World War II to leave us a better world, free from tyranny, so we could enjoy the benefits of democracy. It is our generation's responsibility not to leave the burden of cancer and other serious diseases to our children."

At the Summit, 250 leaders of the cancer movement developed action plans aimed at accelerating cures. U.S. Senator Jay Rockefeller spoke about the need for wider access to cancer therapies for all Americans. Then Milken delivered one of the most important speeches of his career calling for a "rethinking" of the War on Cancer that would move it from a "war of attrition" to a "plan of attack." He outlined a ten-point plan:

1. Internationalize the war on cancer;
2. Invest more;
3. Recruit a world-class scientific team;
4. Coordinate worldwide cancer resources;
5. Accelerate technology transfers;
6. Push the technological envelope;
7. Create a "world library of organic chemicals";
8. Accelerate approval of new drugs;
9. Get product to market faster;
10. Mobilize patients and families.

The speech (see Appendix C) concluded with an emotional appeal:

"We have strived to leave our children a world devoid of war, yet more American lives will be lost in one year to cancer than were lost in all the wars of this century.

"We have strived to leave our children with a country free from debt, yet we are burdening them with massive medical costs associated with an aging population and ever-increasing rates of cancer.

"We have strived to leave our children with a world that celebrates and cherishes the sanctity of a single human life, yet we are unwilling to make the financial and moral commitments necessary to lift the burden of cancer from the next generation.

"Through sins of omission as well as commission, we have created a world where one in five will have their lives cut short by cancer. This is too great a burden to leave to our children and grandchildren.

"For those children and the children of future generations, let us find a cure for cancer. Let us do it now.

"Let us choose life."

Among those who listened to the speech was the new director of the National Cancer Institute, Richard Klausner, M.D., who was joined at the Summit by every living former NCI director. Klausner had already reviewed the white paper from the previous summer's Working Meeting on Standards and now he had evidence of growing support for faster action. Soon he was on the phone to President Clinton's healthcare advisors in the White House.

Early in 1996, the President signed an Executive Order that revised the FDA's review process for experimental cancer drugs to make them more quickly available to patients. "The waiting is over," said Clinton. "We cannot guarantee miracles, but at least now hope is on the way."

Although the PCF is not a lobbying organization, it worked with other patient-advocacy groups to raise awareness in Washington of the potential benefits for patients that might result from streamlining laws and regulations affecting medical research. In 1997, Congress passed The FDA Modernization Act, which sought to reduce the average time required for drug review, streamlined the approval process for drug manufacturing changes, codified regulations to increase patient access to experimental drugs, and provided for an expanded patient-accessible database on clinical trials.

Several of the recommendations promoted by the PCF and many other organizations in the mid-1990s – greater investment, better coordinated resources, accelerated technology transfers, a library of organic chemical compounds and faster drug approvals – have been implemented or are part of the "roadmap for medical research" that NIH Director Dr. Elias Zerhouni sent Congress in 2003. Among other initiatives, the "roadmap" would:

- Promote interdisciplinary groups of scientists;
- Translate discoveries from the lab to the clinic faster;
- Establish a public collection of chemical compounds;
- Give patients swifter access to new drugs.

It's show time

As pointed out in Chapter 11, scientists are increasingly convinced that lifestyle decisions play a significant role in most cancers. But genes are also a major factor. The more relatives a man has with prostate cancer, the higher the risk. An example of this correlation can be seen in David Koch's family. Koch, who is executive vice president of Koch Industries, Inc., a leading diversified energy firm and the second-largest privately held company in America, is one of the nation's most prominent philanthropists.

A board member of major medical and educational institutions, including the Prostate Cancer Foundation, Memorial Sloan-Kettering Cancer Center and the Massachusetts Institute of Technology, Koch has contributed time and energy as well as generous financial support to the PCF and cancer research in general (see Chapter 9). Koch and all three of his brothers have been diagnosed with prostate cancer.

For many years, researchers have tried to recruit such families with a high incidence of prostate cancer to participate in genetic research studies. But it hasn't been easy to find them. In ten years of trying, The Johns Hopkins School of Medicine had been able to recruit only 90 such families. In 1995, Dr. Paul Lange, chief of urology at the University of Washington, whose gene-research work had been supported by the PCF, explained the problem to Milken, who had an idea. Back in the early 1980s, he had arranged the financing that allowed media entrepreneur Ted Turner to expand CNN, the Cable News Network. Now maybe CNN could return the favor.

Milken called Larry King, a longtime friend whose *Larry King Live* reached a nationwide audience every night, and explained that the CNN show could encourage families to sign up for genetic studies. King wasn't enthusiastic. *"It doesn't sound like a very exciting broadcast concept, Mike. We've never done a show like that on cancer. It's too negative. People will tune out. Maybe you should talk to Ted. If he says OK, I'll do it."* Turner approved the show after Milken promised to assemble a first-rate panel of guests.

On November 13, 1995, the night before the Cancer Summit, King interviewed Milken, General Norman Schwarzkopf (who had recently been diagnosed with prostate cancer), Skip Holden and Leroy Hood, M.D., Ph.D. One of the world's leading scientists, Dr. Hood is the inventor of the DNA gene sequencer, which is the technological foundation for contemporary molecular biology. He is the author of more than 500 peer-reviewed papers, co-founder of several biotechnology companies, holder of a dozen patents, winner of the Lasker Award for studies of immune diversity, and the author of textbooks in biochemistry, immunology, biology and genetics.

Hood explained a new initiative called PROGRESS, the name of a PCF-funded Prostate Cancer Genetic Research Study that he would lead at the University of Washington and the Fred Hutchinson Cancer Research Center. Following the broadcast, more than 3,000 people from 18 countries called the program to learn more about the study. As a result, nearly 300 families with three or more close relatives with prostate cancer were recruited for gene studies. Dr. Hood explained the scientific benefit:

"In funding the initial development of the study and the associated molecular and statistical analysis, the Prostate Cancer Foundation took a major step forward in advancing our knowledge of the genetic causes of prostate cancer. PCF funds allowed the initial contacts with hundreds of prostate cancer families to be made; baseline data and DNA samples to be collected; and DNA samples from members of these families to be genotyped with markers that span the human genome. Information about the types of genes important in this disease is likely to play an important role in the development of targeted therapeutics."

It's not just men

Many of the most active advocates in the cancer war are women. Milken points out that when he speaks about medical topics – even prostate cancer – to audiences where 90 percent of the seats are filled by men, at least half the questions come from the 10 percent who are women. Ellen Stovall, executive director of the NCCS, has been a strong voice for patients for many years. Lori Milken has been active as PCF vice president and a board member from the beginning. Cindy Crawford has appeared on national television to discuss the links between nutrition and cancer. Lynda Resnick (see Chapter 9) has been tireless in her efforts on behalf of the PCF. Other PCF board members making important contributions include Helene Brown, Sue Gin, Lorraine Spurge and Elaine Wynn.

Financial journalist and author Beth Kobliner began to take an active role in the search for a prostate cancer cure when her father was diagnosed in 1997. She contributed to the PCF newsletter and website and has made frequent appeals to members of Congress and the President for a greater commitment to research funding.

Sue Gin, a PCF board member and businesswoman, learned that three of her employees had prostate cancer within a few weeks in 1996. *"All of a sudden, the disease was right at my doorstep,"* she recalls. The more she learned about the disease, the more she realized that it affects families and communities, not just individual men. In 1997, Gin was part of a White House roundtable discussion on national issues. *"I told President Clinton that the government and the community need to give prostate cancer a higher profile,"* she says.

On a roll

All this activity was quickly bringing prostate cancer into greater public awareness. Hardly a day passed that some publication wasn't calling the PCF requesting an interview about this previously little-known threat to men. Many of the reporters had scant knowledge of the disease, however. Of even greater concern was the fact that there was only sporadic coverage of the entire cancer field even though one of every four Americans dies from one of its various forms. Milken decided to meet with Walter Isaacson, then the managing editor of *Time* magazine. "Walter," he said, *"You have war correspondents covering every conflict around the world. But you don't have a correspondent covering the biggest war here at home, the War on Cancer."* Isaacson agreed to consider increased coverage.

Some months later, *Time's* Leon Jaroff was on the phone. *"We'd like to do a cover story about prostate cancer and put you on the cover."* Milken appreciated the fact that a major magazine finally had realized the importance of prostate cancer. And he was happy to tell his story. But he suggested that a cover photo of a war hero like General Schwarzkopf would draw more readers.

Within weeks of the Schwarzkopf cover story in the spring of 1996, PCF board member Andy Grove, chairman of Intel Corporation, told the story of his prostate cancer treatment in *Time's* sister publication, *Fortune* magazine. Grove was candid about the agonizing decisions prostate cancer patients face, the potential for sexual side effects, and the need for patients to assert themselves in interviewing different medical specialists. Clearly prostate cancer was coming out of the closet.

All the publicity helped to increase public knowledge of the disease and build a constituency for increased Federal research funding. But something more was needed to make sure that broad constituency was heard loud and clear on Capitol Hill. Something big.

"No More Cancer!"

It was one of those days that remind you why, in the time before air conditioning, Washington, D.C. virtually shut down in the summer. The humidity got a head start into the 90s early in the morning; but the temperature soon passed it. And the sun was unrelenting. In short, it was a perfect day. Perfect because 150,000 people representing 600 cancer organizations had gathered on The National Mall to raise the profile of cancer. Hundreds of thousands more rallied in 200 cities across America that Saturday, September 26, 1998. But it was the group on The Mall that aimed their chants of "No More Cancer!" just a few hundred yards east toward the dome of the U.S. Capitol.

And it was a turning point. Since that day in 1998, Congress has doubled the federal investment in cancer research.

They called it "THE MARCH: Coming Together to Conquer Cancer," a sincere, if unwieldy, name for the maturing of the anti-cancer movement. Taking a cue from the AIDS activists of the 1980s, the previously staid collection of cancer advocacy organizations coalesced into a national force that could not be ignored.

The roots of this extraordinary event reached back three years to November 1995 during the National Cancer Summit. PCF executives met with Ellen Stovall, executive director of the NCCS, the cancer survivorship group, and Amy Langer, head of the Breast Cancer Alliance. Milken, who had been stressing the idea that the cancer community should work together rather than pit one disease against another, remembers the meeting:

"As the Prostate Cancer Foundation had begun establishing a public persona, we delivered the message that we and other cancer groups were on the same team. We were asking for a dramatic increase in cancer funding at the NCI, and had begun to reach out to groups such as the National Coalition for Cancer Survivorship which, at the time, didn't even have a computer or a secretary. The PCF began to help provide some of that infrastructure. As we increased our fund-raising capabilities, we learned that other foundations were having trouble raising money. That's why it was so important to stress that we were standing together."

No more tuning out

The leaders of all the cancer organizations had left the 1995 Cancer Summit pledging to stay in touch and coordinate more of their future efforts. A few months later, in February 1996, Milken again appeared on CNN's *Larry King Live* to discuss nutrition and cancer. Chatting with King after the show, he suggested a future show focusing on the lives of cancer survivors and their growing assertiveness in demanding more action in the War on Cancer. King readily agreed – after the positive public response to the previous November's show on the genetics of cancer, he no longer feared that the subject would make viewers tune out.

Meanwhile NCI Director Richard Klausner had asked cancer activist Ellen Sigal, Ph.D., a member of the NCI's Board of Scientific Advisors, to coordinate activities commemorating the 25th anniversary of the National Cancer Act. Sigal had been having conversations with the PCF's new executive director, Richard ("Rick") Atkins, M.D., about ideas for "mobilizing Congress," a theme she cited in a letter to Milken:

"Michael, I believe we can really make a difference. We share the same objectives and I would be delighted if we could work together on this goal that we both have so much passion for. The anniversary could be used to reach a large public audience who would mobilize Congress into action. You have already made

a major impact and I have no doubt that with your commitment and passion we can make all of this a reality."

During the summer of 1996, Milken joined with philanthropist and industrialist Jon M. Huntsman, also a cancer survivor, to form the National Prostate Cancer Coalition (NPCC), an umbrella organization of survivor groups, research scientists, clinicians, associations and foundations. The NPCC's goal was to develop and implement a comprehensive advocacy agenda for prostate cancer, to reach out to at-risk communities, and to give smaller advocacy groups a voice. Soon they had organized their constituent groups to start collecting hundreds of thousands of signatures on a petition to Congress for increased research funding.

On April 7, 1997, *Larry King Live* featured Milken; Ellen Stovall of the NCCS; ABC News commentator and cancer survivor Sam Donaldson; CBS [now CNN] news anchor and breast-cancer activist Paula Zahn; talk show host and cancer survivor Morton Downey Jr.; and actor Robert Urich, also a cancer survivor. (Downey and Urich have since passed away.) After each guest had talked about the need for action, King confronted the entire group asking, "Why don't you form an army of cancer survivors and march on Washington, D.C. to demand a cure for cancer?"

"Mad as Hell"

Although the idea of an event had been percolating since the 1995 Cancer Summit, that challenge from King helped focus the cancer advocacy community on the idea of a massive demonstration. Over the summer of 1997, the PCF's Rick Atkins worked closely with Stovall to line up more organizations behind the concept of "an army of cancer survivors." It would be a true grass-roots movement. They wanted all the different cancer organizations to get to know each other better so they would become a more-cohesive political force – a phenomenon that had been proven by the breast cancer movement, which had brought dozens of scattered groups under a unified umbrella.

On October 23rd, Milken, Stovall and Sam Donaldson returned to *Larry King Live* along with model Cindy Crawford, whose brother died of leukemia; tennis star and children's cancer advocate Andrea Jaeger; and figure skating champion Scott Hamilton, who had survived testicular cancer. They used the opportunity to announce a March on Washington the following September. During the program, General Norman Schwarzkopf, a prostate cancer survivor and hero of the 1991 Gulf War, called in to offer support. He was named honorary chairman of the March.

Schwarzkopf was blunt: *"When the American people see how woefully underfunded cancer research is, they will be mad as hell. I'm going to be at the March and I challenge every other cancer survivor and every other American to be there with me."*

These were stirring words; but it takes a lot of money to organize 600 groups and half a million people in 200 cities for a coordinated and effective effort. Estimates of the cost ranged from five to ten million dollars. The situation reminded Milken of 1993, when he kick-started the growth of prostate cancer research with a $25-million grant from the Milken Family Foundation rather than wait until enough smaller contributions had been collected. Now, in 1997, he was too impatient to wait for hundreds of organizations to gear up their fund-raising even though the March was designed to be a grass-roots movement. So he persuaded fellow PCF board member Sidney Kimmel, founder and chairman of the Jones Apparel Group and a longtime philanthropist, to join him in committing most of the money needed to assure that the March would go forward. Smaller contributions came in later from several pharmaceutical and biotechnology companies and other groups.

Coast to Coast

During the months leading up to the March, Atkins and Stovall recruited the "army," bringing together hundreds of cancer groups, plus survivors, scientists, government officials, healthcare providers and other concerned citizens. With the growing use of the Internet, word quickly spread across the country that something very important was going to happen on the National Mall in September 1998.

The PCF and other groups were determined, however, that the March should be more than a single day of quickly forgotten demonstrations. An integral part of the planning was to create an ongoing program that would help accelerate cancer research. This research arm of the March was led by Dr. Anna Barker, a scientist and corporate executive who later became Deputy Director of the National Cancer Institute for Strategic Scientific Initiatives. Barker headed an influential study of what needed to be changed in the cancer research process to get faster results, especially in the way clinical trials were conducted. This effort was part of the groundwork for the NCI's pioneering Leadership Roundtable meeting in January 2004 (see Chapter 14). Today, Dr. Barker is one of the leading proponents of interagency programs that can optimize the development and review processes for new cancer drugs and technologies.

By bike and by bus

Early in July 1998, breast cancer survivor Dani Grady of San Diego started "Conquer Cancer Coast to Coast," an 11-week, 3,600-mile bicycle ride across the U.S. Joined by other riders along the way, Grady planned to lead the group onto the Mall during the September 26th march. Other activists helped organize local rallies, marches, town hall meetings and vigils in cities across the country. Governors and mayors issued proclamations of survivor days.

On July 15th, a large, PCF-sponsored van pulled up to the east front of the U.S. Capitol to offer prostate-cancer and breast-cancer screenings to members of Congress. Aside from the public service of the screenings, it turned out to be an effective way to raise the PCF profile. As luck would have it, a rare joint session of Congress was held that day to hear a speech by the visiting President of Romania. Most members of Congress and many of their spouses attended, assuring a steady flow of visitors to the van. First in line was Ann Simpson, the wife of former Wyoming Senator Alan Simpson. Each visitor received literature about plans for the March on September 26th.

Beginning on September 25th, marchers across the eastern half of the U.S. piled onto buses bound for Washington. (One devoted busload of women from Alabama traveled 14 hours non-stop, attended the Cancer March all day, and then turned around to return home.)

Early that Friday evening, Vice President Al Gore and Tipper Gore held a reception for several hundred March organizers and participants in a tent on the grounds of the Naval Observatory, the Vice Presidential residence. Gore invited Milken, Atkins, Kimmel, Stovall and a few others into the residence to discuss the event and he soon agreed to speak the next day.

An inextinguishable candle

Later, as the sun eased below the western end of the Mall, tens of thousands of cancer survivors gathered at the Lincoln Memorial for a candlelight vigil to honor the memory of those who had lost their lives to cancer. After an interfaith service, there were brief speeches by General Schwarzkopf, Scott Hamilton, Andrea Jaeger and other celebrities. Following a musical performance, the Reverend Jesse Jackson rose to speak. He began softly, then gradually raised his booming voice to exhort the gathering:

> "Music is a universal sound that gets our attention. Cancer is a universal pain that wipes out lives. And yet dreamers will not surrender to cancer. WE WILL OUT-DREAM, OUT-WORK, OUT-RESEARCH, OUT-FIGHT! We will conquer cancer because our minds are made up. Tonight we march for public policy, new priorities; we march for our basic rights, the right to live, the right to breathe, the right to build, the right to grow, the right to family."

Other moving comments came from less-famous March participants. As people stood holding candles, one woman said she was a survivor of more than 10 reoccurrences of cancer, but she believed she was "a candle that cannot be extinguished."

The next morning, more than 100,000 more people arrived, most by bus, and crowded onto the Mall. Helene Brown, a PCF board member, honorary life member of the American Cancer Society, and self-described "political oncologist" at UCLA's Jonsson Comprehensive Cancer Center, turned to PCF executive director Rick Atkins. *"I told you for months this event was going to backfire, that it would never happen because you were dealing with a motherhood and apple-pie issue – people don't congregate around motherhood and apple pie. I have just one thing to tell you – I was wrong."*

The Mall was dotted with white tents housing cancer education and prevention displays. In one tent, several of the speakers and performers autographed a poster commemorating the March. In addition to Mike Milken, the signers included former U.S. Senator and presidential nominee Bob Dole; and recording artist Graham Nash of the group Crosby, Stills & Nash. Milken later recalled the irony:

> *"Think back to 1969. A young Robert Dole from Kansas is giving his maiden speech in the U.S. Senate, the ultimate bastion of American tradition. That same year, Graham Nash, with defiant long hair, is performing at Woodstock before a crowd of half-dressed young people bent on strengthening a counterculture opposed to the Establishment that Dole represents. Dole had won two purple hearts in World War II; the Woodstock crowd vehemently opposed the Vietnam War. But there was Nash on the Mall telling me, 'I never thought I'd be in such agreement with Senator Dole, much less signing the same document.'"*

King Hussein of Jordan, who would lose his life to cancer just a few months later, had planned to speak but was not well enough to do so. His wife, Queen Noor, attended to him in a VIP tent.

Other tents provided ice water and shelter from the heat for the marchers. Some were staffed by oncology nurses and doctors.

Children were not forgotten amid all the serious events. In one corner of the Mall, kids were enjoying a supervised play area with face painting and other games. Most memorably, a Children's Wall near Constitution Avenue, built at Milken's request as a memorial to cancer's youngest victims, was filled with poignant remembrances – a favorite toy, a good-bye poem, a pair of tiny sneakers or a picture of a loved one. Little children came and brought remembrances of a brother or sister lost too soon. Almost everyone who stopped at the wall walked away in tears.

Let's take the Hill!

As the formal program began under a baking noonday sun, Vice President Gore tossed his suit jacket aside, rolled up his sleeves and told the crowd, *"We want to be the generation that wins the war on cancer. Some people still say it is impossible to find a cure. A hundred years ago, people said the same thing about smallpox."*

"We've established a beachhead," said Senator Tom Harkin of Iowa; then he turned and pointed up at the U.S. Capitol. *"Now we have to take the Hill!"* Emphasizing that sentiment, representatives of the National Prostate Cancer Coalition announced that they were delivering 750,000 signatures urging Congress to increase research funding.

Stressing a grander message, PCF board member and former Los Angeles Rams football star Rosey Grier shouted, *"If we use our voices together, we can start a mighty roar that will be heard worldwide."*

After pedaling across the Mall – the last lap of her cross-country ride – an excited Dani Grady bounded up the steps of the speakers' platform hoisting her bicycle over her head. *"I've been waiting a long time to say this – Hello Washington! Hello America!"* Then, echoing Henry V at Agincourt, she added, *"Remember where you were today."*

Singer Aretha Franklin electrified the audience with some gospel and soul standards, then promptly sat down and wrote a $15,000 check to help with the March expenses.

The crowd greeted speaker after speaker – Schwarzkopf, Tipper Gore, Queen Noor, Senator Connie Mack, ABC political analyst Cokie Roberts, Sam Donaldson and several more – with chants of "No More Cancer!" and "Yes, We Can!" At the side of the platform, an American Sign Language interpreter signed the speakers' words for the hearing impaired.

Then the PCF chairman moved to the microphones. "My name is Mike Milken and I am a cancer survivor." The crowd yelled encouragement while one group near the front hoisted placards reading FAMILIES FIGHTING PROSTATE CANCER. *"You make history today,"* Milken continued. *"Today we are united to defeat cancer. Today in Washington we think back to our parents, our grandparents and generations of Americans who fought to make this country free and give us a better life. We think back to generations of Americans and scientists who have rid us of smallpox and polio. My father had polio but he died from cancer. It's our commitment today that our children will not remember cancer. For those children and the children of future generations, let's get on with finding a cure for cancer and let's do it now."*

Dr. Joel Nelson, a prominent urologist, was one of several Johns Hopkins doctors who brought their families from Baltimore to be part of the March. "It's not often that you're involved in something that has that kind of magnitude. As a scientist and physician who takes care of patients with cancer, I was really inspired. It made me think about what we're capable of. I knew then that all that stands between us and success is ourselves saying, 'Let's get going.' That's what the March was all about."

The PCF played a leadership role in organizing The March: Coming Together to Conquer Cancer. In September 1998, 150,000 people representing 600 cancer organizations gathered on the National Mall in Washington to demand increased federal funding for cancer research. Hundreds of thousands more rallied in 200 cities across America. In the five years after The March, federal funding of cancer research increased nearly 70 percent.

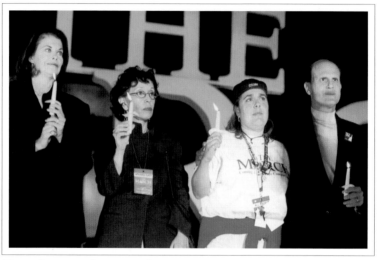

Sherry Lansing, chairman of Paramount Pictures Motion Picture Group (left); Ellen Sigal, Ph.D., founder and chairperson of Friends of Cancer Research (second from left); and Mike Milken join a young marcher at a Lincoln Memorial candlelight vigil the night before The March to remember those who had died from cancer.

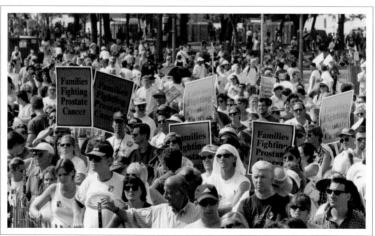

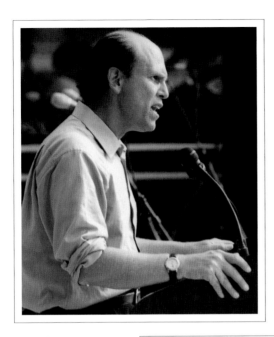

"It is our commitment today that our children will not remember cancer. For those children and the children of future generations, let's get on with finding a cure for cancer and let's do it now."

Mike Milken

"I've been waiting a long time to say this — Hello Washington! Hello America! Remember where you were today."

Breast cancer survivor Dani Grady after riding her bicycle across the country from San Diego.

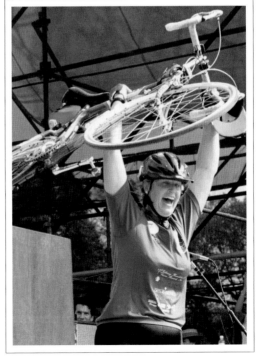

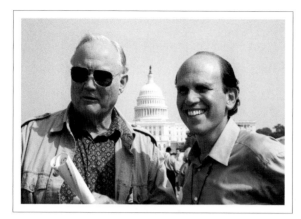

General Norman Schwarzkopf and Mike Milken at The March. Schwarzkopf said, *"When the American people see how woefully underfunded cancer research is, they will be mad as hell."*

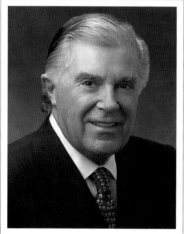

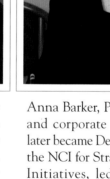

Longtime philanthropist Sidney Kimmel joined with Mike Milken to provide the majority of funding for the event. Kimmel has funded cancer research centers across the U.S., including Baltimore, New York, Philadelphia and San Diego.

Anna Barker, Ph.D., a scientist and corporate executive who later became Deputy Director of the NCI for Strategic Scientific Initiatives, led the effort to harness the energy created by The March and accelerate the cancer research process.

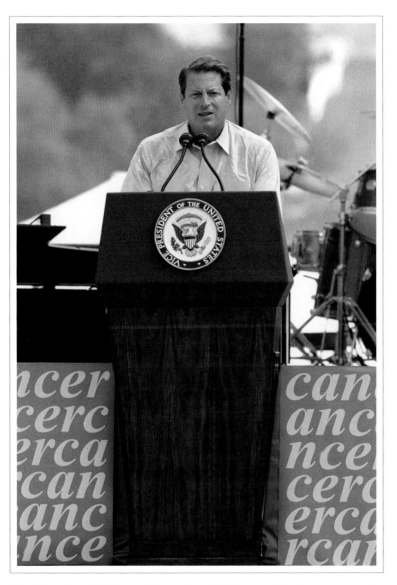

Vice President Al Gore told marchers: *"We want to be the generation that wins the war on cancer. Some people still say it's impossible to find a cure. A hundred years ago, people said that about smallpox."*

Keeping it going

The effects of the March are still being felt. In less than a year, Milken was invited to testify about cancer funding before the U.S. Senate Subcommittee on Labor, Health & Human Services and Education Appropriations. He asked Joe Torre, the manager of the New York Yankees, who had recently been diagnosed with prostate cancer, if he'd also like to make a statement to the committee. It was June, the middle of baseball season, and Torre couldn't be away from the team for long.

Milken agreed to pick up Torre in the morning at his suburban New York home and fly him to Washington, getting him back to Yankee Stadium for that night's game. On the flight to Washington, Milken was reviewing his prepared remarks with an aide. *"I don't think these numbers are right,"* said Milken. *"You see here where it compares cancer funding to the gross domestic product? There should be another zero after the decimal point."*

Torre, who was munching on a bagel across the aisle, looked pained. *"Geez, Mike, I don't know about those numbers. All I know about math is if I have more than nine guys on the field, I'm in big trouble!"*

Later that day, Milken and Torre were joined by former Senator Bob Dole. All three testified before the committee chaired by Senator Arlen Specter of Pennsylvania. Milken reminded the committee about the previous year's March:

> *"How much firepower do we need to defeat cancer? Last fall, as part of 'The March ... Coming Together to Conquer Cancer,' I suggested to Senators Connie Mack and Dianne Feinstein, at a hearing of the Senate Cancer Caucus, that the annual federal investment in cancer research be increased to $10 billion. That's less than $40 per American. It is a fraction of the cost of failure – the cost of treating the more than 100 million Americans currently living who are expected to get cancer.*

"I believe that we can accelerate science. If we give cancer researchers the same kinds of tools that technology companies employ in accelerating scientific development, we can find a cure faster. We have talented people working on this inside and outside the government. Let's give them the tools and the incentives to finish this job. Let's send a message to our best and brightest young scientists that cancer research is an exciting profession. Finally, let's show all these dedicated people that we share their sense of urgency."

Funding the future

Not long after The March, Milken hosted a meeting at Lake Tahoe to help coordinate the activities of several major funders of prostate cancer research – the National Cancer Institute, the Department of Defense, the American Cancer Society, the PCF and others. This led to a "Funders Conference" at the NCI in Washington that was attended by Richard Klausner, then the Director of the NCI; Andy Grove; Milken; Skip Holden; Rick Atkins; government officials from other agencies; and business executives representing major health sciences companies. This meeting and similar conferences over the next several years helped refine the NCI's prostate cancer strategy. It has been a novel and effective way to improve coordination of public and private efforts to advance research on an individual disease.

"A Brilliant String"

When the Dallas Cowboys are preparing to play the New York Giants, the two head coaches don't sit down in advance and explain their game plans to each other. On game day, there will be one winner and one loser. To avoid becoming the loser, each team guards its playbooks like the gold in Fort Knox.

Unfortunately, researchers at major medical centers have too often followed something like the football strategy, fearing that if they share the interim results of their work, they might lose credit for breakthrough ideas before they can be published in prestigious journals. They also worry that they will be embarrassed if the final results are not as strong as suggested earlier. And they are concerned that others might take their preliminary work in different directions. While these are legitimate concerns, Milken felt that there was room for more coordination across institutions:

> "If scientists are working on the same problem in different cities, they should share their findings. That will accelerate science and shorten the path to cures so that everyone wins, especially patients."

The Prostate Cancer Foundation's first priority had been to seed the field of cancer research by getting funds out to scientists quickly, with no bureaucratic delays. This could speed progress and attract the best new researchers to the field. But as Dr. Andrew von Eschenbach, Director of the National Cancer Institute, notes in the Foreword to this book, "There was a string attached, a brilliant string." As a condition of receiving PCF funding, each researcher would be required to report on his or her work in front of hundreds of peers from other institutions at an annual scientific retreat.

Mix it up

As with the Call-to-Action dinners in Washington, the PCF tried to provide real recognition to the award winners. They wanted the retreats to be located in a pleasant or inspiring location away from big-city distractions. The first two PCF Scientific Retreats were held overlooking the Pacific Ocean at the historic Biltmore Hotel in Santa Barbara, California. Later, they would move to an even more dramatic setting on the shores of Lake Tahoe near the Nevada-California border. The goal was not just interaction among academicians, but also to have these non-profit scientists mix with their commercial counterparts:

"When I went to that conference at M.D. Anderson after I was diagnosed," said Milken, *"I didn't see any interaction with for-profit companies. I felt that it was important to get them working together. No government science center has ever brought a product to market by itself, and I wanted to make sure the biotech and pharmaceutical industries were focused on prostate cancer. Gordon Binder [then chairman of Amgen, the world's largest biotechnology company] had told me that there wasn't enough work in basic science for a company like Amgen to devote a major portion of its research program to cancer.*

"I wanted to make a statement that we were going to deal with prostate cancer and that these researchers weren't second-class citizens. At our first Scientific Retreat, everyone sat in their own groups: the M.D. Anderson doctors sat at one table, Hopkins at another, and the biotech people were across the room. At the time, there was a feeling that for-profit research was beneath and behind work done in the university setting. It wasn't until the second day, with the presentations from some of the leaders in the biotech firms, that everyone began to mingle. All of sudden, respect was being established and people were realizing how they could help each other. It became obvious that they all needed to interact."

Most participants in the early Scientific Retreats were oncologists and other clinicians, with a smattering of representatives from pharmaceutical and biotechnology companies. Each year, the event grew in size and importance – 100 participants in 1994, 130 in 1995, 200 by 1996 and so on until by 2003 the PCF had to cut off registrations at 350 to maintain a collaborative atmosphere. Although oncologists still comprise the largest group of attendees, the Retreat has become more diverse as it has grown. After several years, the agenda included, among others, presentations and participation by epidemiologists, biologists, physicists, chemists, mathematicians, computer scientists, nutrition experts, ethicists, political leaders, investors and investment bankers/analysts who follow the commercial companies working on cancer treatments.

> *"I've been lucky enough to be one of the few analysts who have spoken at the Scientific Retreat to give the Wall Street view in terms of what investors are thinking,"* says Mark Simon, managing director of Citigroup's healthcare unit. *"Over the past ten years, the Prostate Cancer Foundation has built a very powerful brand name for scientific and clinical excellence, such that commercial entities view research funding or research involvement from the PCF as a major validation."*

Many business leaders were invited to the Retreats, especially when they had specific experience that could help accelerate medical science. For example, Martin Wygod first attended in 1995. Wygod, who now heads WebMD, had founded Medco, the nation's leading pharmacy benefits manager, which handles hundreds of millions of prescriptions annually. Over the years, Wygod contributed useful insights about handling large amounts of data, a process of increasing relevance in medical research.

The PCF Scientific Retreats have been a forum for leading medical scientists. Nobel laureate Andrew Schally, M.D., Ph.D., professor of medicine at Tulane University, has spoken several times. And there have been many important presentations on advanced work in the field. In 1996, Judah Folkman, M.D., professor of cell biology at Harvard Medical School, reported preliminary results of clinical trials using a new generation of anti-angiogenesis drugs designed to close off the blood supply to tumors. The following year, an article in the *Journal of the American Medical Association* said, the *"[PCF's] annual scientific retreat and the research efforts reported there arguably are unique in this nation's history of cancer studies ... [The PCF] seems to be opening the largest single front of the war on cancer."*

Late-night progress

Skip Holden, the PCF medical director, feels the Retreats have become "the premier meeting in the prostate cancer field." Informal discussions at the Retreat often continue well past midnight.

One of those discussions in 1996 presaged major changes in the research program of the University of California at San Francisco (UCSF). The PCF assembled a group that included the University's chancellor, the head of its urology department and several of its biomedical researchers, Intel Chairman Andy Grove, and the Lieutenant Governor of California. Howard Soule, Ph.D., the PCF scientific director, recalls the meeting:

> *"We sequestered ourselves for several hours to evaluate UCSF, a cancer center with enormous potential that wasn't doing enough. At the time, UCSF had a fabulous basic science component, but people in research weren't working with those in the clinics. Their clinical research was only so-so, but the intellectual content and talent to be successful were there."*

Milken made the same point to the UCSF contingent that he had made at Harvard in 1993 – their future as a cancer center was at risk if their major donors went to other medical centers for treatment. While that would surely mean fewer major contributions, there would be a more serious consequence: their best researchers and clinicians would abandon UCSF for other institutions. Then Milken offered the resources of the PCF and its board of directors to help UCSF get back on track.

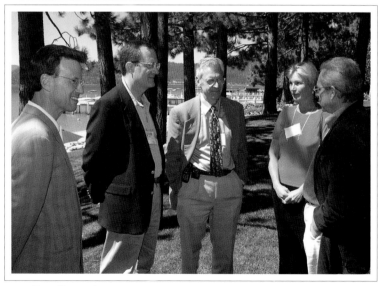

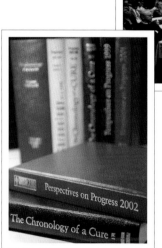

Each year, the Prostate Cancer Foundation's Scientific Retreat hosts more than 300 of the world's leading scientists, physicians, biotechnology and pharmaceutical company representatives and government officials. The PCF requires research award winners to present their findings, which are then published in annual volumes.

Lowell Milken, chairman of the Milken Family Foundation (left) at the 2001 PCF Scientific Retreat at Lake Tahoe with (left to right) George Wilding, M.D.; John Wiley, Ph.D., chancellor of the University of Wisconsin; Mrs. Wiley; and PCF Medical Director Stuart Holden, M.D.

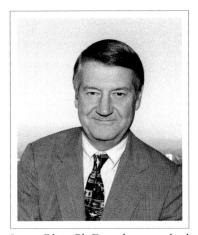

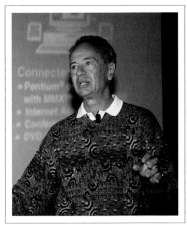

James Blair, Ph.D., a distinguished life sciences researcher and venture capitalist, has helped the PCF integrate successful business principles from high-tech industries with promising research ideas.

Andy Grove, the chairman of Intel and a Prostate Cancer Foundation board member, has worked closely with the PCF to encourage biotechnology and pharmaceutical companies to expand their investment in prostate cancer drugs.

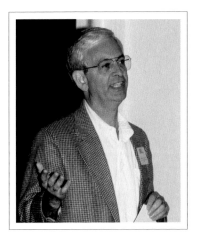

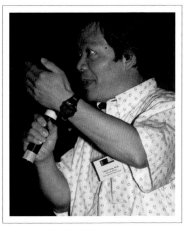

William Catalona, M.D. (left) and Leland Chung, Ph.D., were among the 100 researchers, business leaders and government officials who attended the PCF's first Scientific Retreat in Santa Barbara, California, in 1994. Catalona is now director of the clinical prostate cancer program at Northwestern University. Chung, at Emory University, helps oversee a $10 million grant from the U.S. Department of Defense Prostate Cancer Research Program for a 'Manhattan Project' addressing prostate cancer.

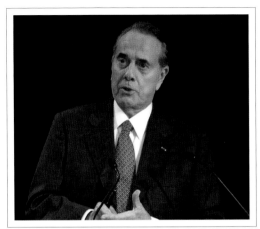

Former U.S. Senator Bob Dole spoke at the 2002 Scientific Retreat. Dole is a longtime PCF supporter, having attended the PCF's first Call-to-Action Dinner in 1993.

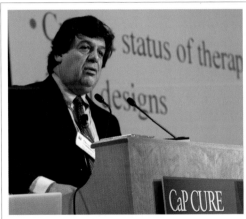

Christopher Logothetis, M.D., who heads the prostate cancer research program at M.D. Anderson Cancer Center, played a key role in developing many new drugs, including Velcade. Logothetis has won multiple PCF research awards.

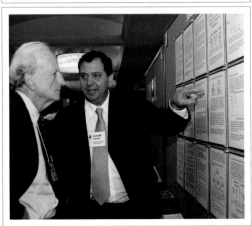

Dr. Gary Becker (left), Nobel laureate in Economics, known for his ground-breaking human capital theories, is a regular participant at the PCF's Scientific Retreats.

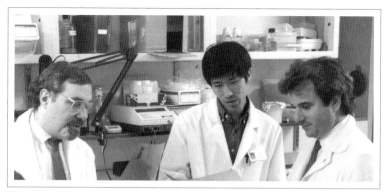

The PCF has always encouraged collaboration between laboratory researchers and clinicians. Neal Rosen, M.D., Ph.D., (left) a cancer researcher, and clinician Howard Scher, M.D. (right), both at Memorial Sloan-Kettering Cancer Center, are collaborating on geldanamycin, a compound that may slow the growth of cancer cells.

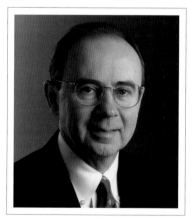

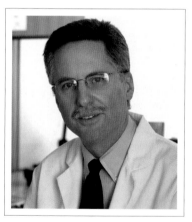

Patrick Walsh, M.D., urologist-in-chief at Johns Hopkins, pioneered nerve-sparing prostate surgery that has led to improved lifestyles for prostate cancer survivors. A frequent participant at Scientific Retreats, he is the author of *Dr. Patrick Walsh's Guide to Surviving Prostate Cancer.*

Peter Carroll, M.D., heads the Urology Department at the University of California, San Francisco, one of eight institutions in the Prostate Cancer Foundation Therapy Consortium.

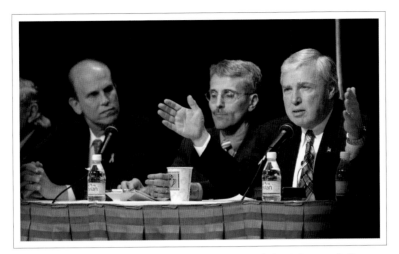

Andrew von Eschenbach, M.D., Director of the National Cancer Institute, speaks at the 2002 Scientific Retreat as PCF Chairman Mike Milken and the Food and Drug Administration's Richard Pazdur listen.

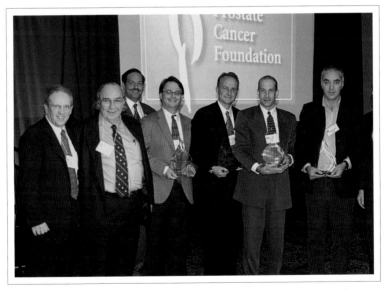

The first Prostate Cancer Foundation Donald S. Coffey Awards were presented at the 2003 PCF Scientific Retreat to Jonathan Simons, M.D.; Joel Nelson, M.D.; Anthony D'Amico, M.D.; and Massimo Loda, M.D. Left to right: PCF Medical Director Stuart "Skip" Holden, M.D.; Donald S. Coffey, Ph.D.; PCF CEO Leslie Michelson; Simons; Nelson; D'Amico; and Loda.

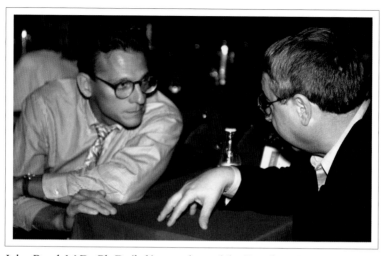

John Reed, M.D., Ph.D. (left), president of the Burnham Institute in San Diego, is a renowned expert on apoptosis, the process by which cells die. Reed's work, supported by the PCF, has become a benchmark in the understanding of apoptosis in all forms of cancer, and his success has helped develop a burgeoning scientific community in San Diego.

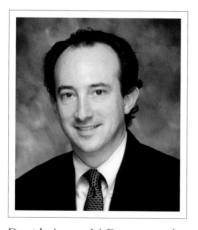

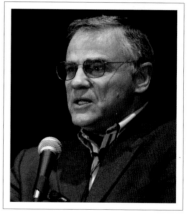

David Agus, M.D., research director of the Louis Warschaw Prostate Cancer Center at Cedars-Sinai Medical Center, is a leading translational researcher who is developing methods to accelerate prostate cancer research.

Leroy Hood, M.D., Ph.D., a frequent participant at Prostate Cancer Foundation Scientific Retreats, is the director of the Institute for Systems Biology.

Dr. Peter Carroll, chairman of the department of urology at UCSF, picks up the story:

> "Mike added focus and urgency, and gave us insight into how to build programs and allocate resources. He's a guy who moves planets into alignment to allow things to happen. Within three years of that 1997 meeting, we got our SPORE grant (see Chapter 5) and established UCSF as one of the premier centers of excellence for prostate cancer research and care in the world. This has culminated in a very big donation that will help build more than 10,000 square feet of new laboratory space for new investigators. We're now able to move the science along faster and deliver greater benefits to many more patients."

Consorting with progress

The PCF's Therapy Consortium brings together researchers at leading medical research centers. The Consortium was formed in 1996 to create new clinical trials, recruit participants and share results to hasten effective new therapies for men with advanced prostate cancer. Members of the Consortium test each other's ideas; collaborate in designing and evaluating clinical trials, many of which are funded by the PCF; and develop new drugs and treatments. It is a respectful, collegial, but challenging relationship that supercedes competition to accelerate science. As of late 2003, members of the Consortium included:

- Cedars-Sinai Medical Center, Los Angeles
- Dana-Farber Cancer Institute at the Harvard Medical School
- The Johns Hopkins University Medical Institutions
- M.D. Anderson Cancer Center at the University of Texas
- Memorial Sloan-Kettering Cancer Center
- University of California, San Francisco
- University of Michigan Comprehensive Cancer Center
- University of Wisconsin Medical School

Annual spending on prostate cancer research at these institutions has grown from $6,420,000 to $73,900,000 in the past decade. The number of scientists and physicians working in their laboratories has grown from 50 to 252 over the same period.

Over several years, the Consortium has acted as a planning group to initiate new academic and industrial trials for prostate cancer treatments; screened new drugs for inclusion in trials; participated in clinical-trial standardization programs; and jointly selected a clinical research informatics system to link the participating centers. Consortium members have also established taxane-based chemotherapy as a treatment option for advanced prostate cancer (see Chapter 12).

Eric Small, M.D., clinical professor of medicine and urology at UCSF, is enthusiastic about the PCF Consortium. *"The best patient care always comes from integrating the most innovative and novel therapeutics with a vigorous research program. Our participation in the Consortium has helped transform us into a top-tier cancer center. We strengthened our research infrastructure to complement the expertise we already had."*

A great partnership

The Therapy Consortium has focused on speeding treatments from the lab to the clinic. For example, at New York's Memorial Sloan-Kettering Cancer Center, a Consortium member, Neal Rosen, M.D., Ph.D., the head of the Molecular Oncogenesis Laboratory, explores signaling pathways within cells that lead to the development of cancers. By understanding how cancer cells receive signals to divide, Dr. Rosen hopes to find agents – "signaling inhibitors" – that block these signals, preventing the cancer cells from dividing and invading healthy adjacent tissues.

Meanwhile, Howard Scher, M.D., chief of Sloan-Kettering's Genitourinary Oncology Service, oversees development of new therapies including monoclonal antibodies, vaccines and drugs that target specific signaling pathways. *"The beauty,"* says the

PCF's Howard Soule, *"is that Neal discovers it in the lab and can then move it to Howard Scher in the clinic immediately. It's a great partnership. This is exemplary of the top cancer centers. It's very powerful."*

Through the Consortium, Soule and Scher also established a working group that includes the National Cancer Institute, the Food and Drug Administration and academic and industry researchers that is developing standardized clinical-trial guidelines for well patients who have rising PSA scores.

In addition to the Therapy Consortium, the Prostate Cancer Foundation has established other collaborative groups aimed at specific issues. The Gene and Family Studies Consortium, headquartered at the University of Washington and the Fred Hutchinson Cancer Research Center in Seattle, was established to coordinate work at multiple sites aimed at developing a more complete understanding of gene expression in disease. Members of the Consortium have adapted a scanner that produces live-action sequential images of gene function in animal models.

Take it to the bank

Researchers need tissue – blood, skin and tumors – to test the effectiveness of various experimental compounds. Very little tissue was available for prostate cancer research when the Prostate Cancer Foundation was started. By 1995, the PCF had convened a Tissue Bank Summit to establish coordinated protocols for harvesting prostate-cancer tissue. Then the PCF helped fund regional tissue banks at Dana Farber Cancer Institute in Boston; M.D. Anderson Cancer Center in Houston; the University of Washington in Seattle; and Washington University in St. Louis. These institutions, and others that joined later, send prostate cancer tissue to researchers around the world.

Collaborative efforts have also been highlighted at the annual Global Conferences of the Milken Institute, an economic think tank. A signature event at these conferences is a panel of Nobel Prize winners discussing medicine and science. Other panels have explored nutrition and cancer, medical research policy, medical and biotechnology investment, and potential breakthroughs in cancer and heart disease discussed by current and former directors of the National Cancer Institute and the Food and Drug Administration.

Whatever the event, the goal has been to get disparate groups communicating with the expectation that novel ideas will emerge, ideas that can have applicability across a broad range of diseases. The Prostate Cancer Foundation has cooperated with many other groups to encourage an increased national commitment in support of all medical research.

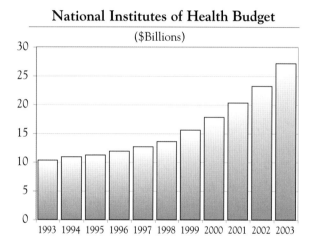

National Institutes of Health Budget

($Billions)

In the five years since "THE MARCH: Coming Together to Conquer Cancer," the budget of the National Cancer Institute devoted to research on all cancers has increased nearly 70 percent.

National Cancer Institute Budget

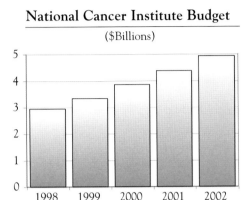

($Billions)

In 2002, after several years of PCF Scientific Retreats at Lake Tahoe, the event moved to Washington, D.C. as a way of reminding public policy leaders that even in the face of a new priority to fight terrorism, progress against disease requires continuous federal research funding.

The 2003 Retreat, also planned for Washington, had to be shifted to New York when Hurricane Isabel virtually shut down the Capital. Speaking in New York, Patrick Walsh, M.D., head of the Brady Urological Institute at Johns Hopkins, began a lecture on the history of prostate cancer surgery by thanking Milken:

> *"You really have made a major contribution to mankind. Among many other accomplishments, you've made prostate cancer a household word."*

Giving of Themselves

*W*hen the Prostate Cancer Foundation was founded in 1993, most Americans knew little about prostate cancer and its devastating effects. Few people realized that some form of cancer strikes one in every two American men and one in three women in their lifetimes; that one in six men would be diagnosed with prostate cancer; or that a man is one-third more likely to develop prostate cancer than a woman is to get breast cancer.

These facts shaped the PCF's strategies for raising funds and raising awareness during its first decade. The initial $25-million grant from a single source (see Chapter 3) got it up and running. But the PCF quickly had to establish a continuing flow of funds from multiple donors and, eventually, from a broad base of public support. PCF executives reached out to potential donors not just for money, but also for the kind of involvement that could dramatically increase public awareness of the disease, and the importance of financing the most promising research.

People won't contribute to a charity just because it's a worthy cause. Something or someone has to make them aware of the need and motivate them to take action. The "something" could be a television broadcast, a local community event or a ceremony during a sports contest. The "someone" is most often a celebrity from the world of entertainment, sports, the arts, politics or business. These are the kinds of personalities who can build awareness, who can really change things.

Fortunately, there is no shortage of high achievers who recognize that their success was built in the context of a free and open society. Many want to give back to that society and are willing to commit their time, talent and money in ways that can help others. Mike Milken was able to leverage his relationships with many of these leaders in their fields – people who had already been active in other charities and could help the PCF cause with their ideas, experience and financial resources.

> "We've reached out to people who are the best in the world at what they do and urged them to get personally involved," says Milken. "We bring these leaders together at events throughout the year so they'll be inspired by each other and get excited about what we're trying to achieve in the laboratory and the clinic. I don't just want them to make a donation or record a 30-second TV spot, although that helps too. I want them to learn what we were doing, to believe in it, and show the world that they believe. That's what motivates the public."

The philanthropists

In a Wall Street career that began in the late 1960s, Milken had financed several thousand companies, many of which are household names today. Collectively, those companies created millions of jobs and contributed mightily to the booming American economy of the late 20th century. Milken knew that the heads of some of these companies he had helped to build maintained a strong interest in medical science. They didn't let him down when he asked them to help. Many pitched in by hosting events in their homes, calling friends to ask for donations, or offering the resources of their businesses in ways that would raise additional funds.

It wasn't just business leaders, however. Entertainment celebrities, sports stars, political figures, well-known artists and television personalities have given valuable time and talent in addition to generous financial support.

Bi-coastal giving

Comedian/actor Bill Cosby and Marshall Cogan hosted the PCF's first major fund-raiser in April 1994 at Cogan's famous 21 Club restaurant in New York. The evening combined celebrities such as Cosby, CNN's Larry King, fashion designer Calvin Klein and football legend Rosey Grier, with leading prostate cancer researchers and many of the people who would soon be among the PCF's most stalwart supporters, including Lynne and Mickey Tarnopol, Leon Black, Claudia and Nelson Peltz, and Martin Wygod.

Just as the festivities were reaching a high point, Grier asked for quiet because he had someone on the speaker phone. Soon, the unmistakable voice of the President of the United States was congratulating the PCF on its contributions to prostate cancer research. Bill Clinton continued:

> "I want to encourage you in what you're doing – getting people in the private sector to work with healthcare folks to find a better way to provide healthcare and to find a cure for prostate cancer. Most of my time has been spent working on breast cancer because my mother had it. But I know how many millions of men have been diagnosed with prostate cancer. So many have lost that fight, but a lot can win. I commend you and the PCF. I'm proud of you. Thank you for what you're doing."

Less than a month later, the PCF hosted an outdoor party in Los Angeles at the glamorous Pickfair Estate, once the home to actors Douglas Fairbanks Jr. and his wife, Mary Pickford. With supporters as diverse as Los Angeles Mayor Richard Riordan (who was later diagnosed with prostate cancer) and Terry Semel, then chairman of Warner Brothers and now chairman of Yahoo!, Pickfair was as great a success on the West Coast as the 21 Club dinner had been in the east. These first two events previewed the substantial fund-raising potential of the Prostate Cancer Foundation.

Soon, major philanthropists such as Ron Perelman, who had long supported breast cancer research, supermarket magnate Ronald Burkle, and Universal CEO Edgar Bronfman pledged major support. Other business leaders who made important contributions included Microsoft's Bill Gates, Cincinnati businessman Carl Lindner, cell phone pioneer Craig McCaw, Viacom's Sumner Redstone and Sun Microsystems CEO Scott McNealy.

What began as a relatively small dinner in a New York restaurant soon developed into a regular event that has become one of the PCF's most successful fund-raisers – the New York Dinner. It was hosted for two years at the Pierre Hotel before moving to the Waldorf Astoria, with its larger ballroom. Guests have been treated to entertainment from such legendary performers as Tony Bennett, Michael Bolton, Cher, Gloria Estefan, Johnny Mathis, Lionel Richie, Paul Simon, Rod Stewart, and Sting, whose father died from prostate cancer. The dinner is now spearheaded by the Tarnopols.

At the 1995 dinner, dubbed "Operation CaP CURE," Gerald Levin, then chairman of Time Warner, introduced General Norman Schwarzkopf, who was honored for his efforts to increase public awareness of prostate cancer. News Corp. Chairman Rupert Murdoch, a prostate cancer survivor who would become one of the largest contributors to the PCF, also attended. Despite the serious cause, the Pierre Hotel's ballroom rocked with laughter as Larry King and Whoopi Goldberg kibitzed their way through their shared duties as masters of ceremonies.

Three years later, nearly 1,200 guests were on hand at the New York Dinner as the PCF launched its PGA SENIOR TOUR for the CURE (now the PGA Champions Tour), featuring a live satellite broadcast with golfing legends Arnold Palmer and Jack Nicklaus playing in Hawaii. Golf fans nationwide pledge money for each birdie notched by their favorite players on the Tour. Senior Tour star Jim Colbert summarized the effect of the public announcement of his prostate cancer diagnosis: *"I couldn't go 100 yards without someone in the gallery saying, 'I had it last year,' 'I had it four years ago,' 'I did the radiation.' It was incredible. Everyone was talking about it. And it was high time."*

Actor Robert Wagner and his actress wife, Jill St. John, hosted the 1999 dinner, which honored New York Yankees manager Joe Torre and longtime PCF supporters Steve and Elaine Wynn. In the

In its first decade, the Prostate Cancer Foundation dramatically increased public awareness of prostate cancer and was able to fund important research projects with the help of hundreds of entertainers, athletes and business leaders, some of whom are shown on the following pages performing or competing at various PCF fund-raising events.

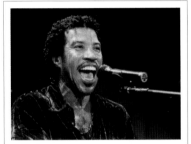

Lionel Richie

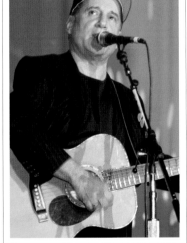

Larry King and
Whoopi Goldberg

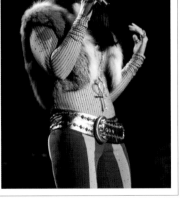

Cher

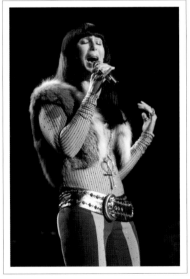

Paul Simon

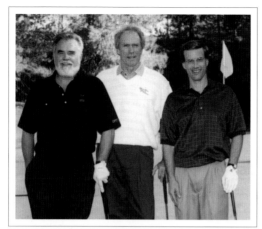

Herb Kohler and Clint Eastwood with Milken Family Foundation Chairman Lowell Milken

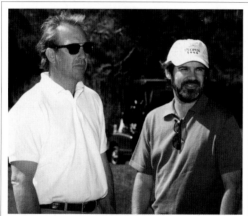

Kevin Costner and Dennis Miller

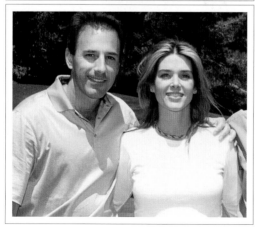

Matt Lauer and Donna Baldwin

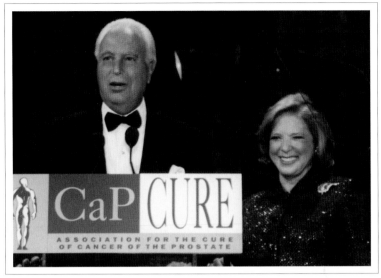

Mickey and Lynne Tarnopol, longtime PCF supporters, have been the driving forces in organizing and hosting the New York Dinners, which have raised millions of dollars for prostate cancer research.

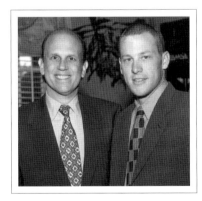

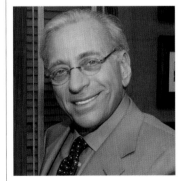

Mike Milken with world-class cyclist Lance Armstrong, who founded the Lance Armstrong Foundation "to enhance the quality of life for those living with, through and beyond cancer."

Businessman Nelson Peltz was one of the first major donors to contribute to the Prostate Cancer Foundation. He attended the first PCF fund-raiser in 1994 at the 21 Club in New York.

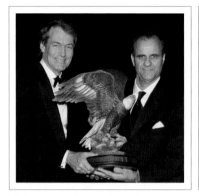

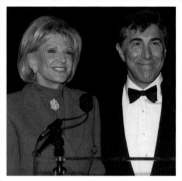

Television host Charlie Rose presents an award to New York Yankees Manager Joe Torre (right) at the PCF's 1999 New York Dinner. Torre, a prostate cancer survivor, has been an active spokesman for the PCF.

Longtime PCF supporters Elaine and Steve Wynn were honored at the 1999 New York Dinner. The Wynns hosted a Las Vegas Invitational golf tournament for several years that raised more than $20 million for the PCF.

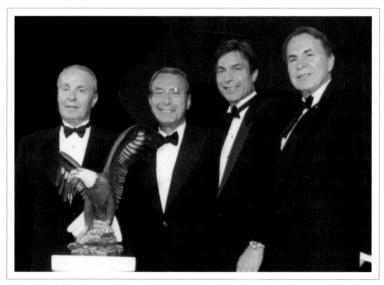

The Mack brothers – David, Bill, Fred and Earle – were honored for their widespread philanthropy and commitment to prostate cancer research at the 2001 New York Dinner.

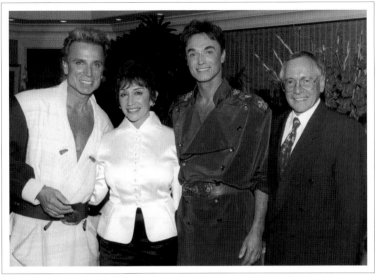

Prostate Cancer Foundation Board Member Lynda Resnick and her husband, Stewart (far right), pictured with Siegfried and Roy at a PCF fund-raising event, have provided a decade of support to the PCF.

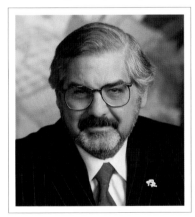

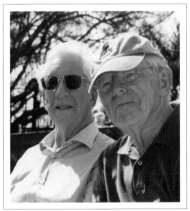

Wine Spectator publisher Marvin Shanken hosts an annual "*A Night to Remember*" dinner to raise funds for the PCF.

Business leaders, Carl Lindner (left) and Charles Dolan, pictured at the Mar-a-Lago fund-raiser, are two of the PCF's strongest supporters. Dolan and his family have also established the Lustgarten Foundation for Pancreatic Cancer Research, adapting several innovative PCF strategies.

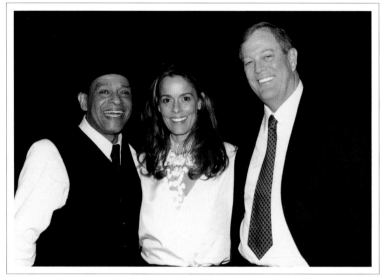

In 2002, the Prostate Cancer Foundation established the David H. Koch Prostate Cancer Research Awards, which have enabled the PCF to provide more than $6 million to fund major research programs at The Johns Hopkins University, The M.D. Anderson Cancer Center, and Memorial Sloan-Kettering Cancer Center. Above, singer Al Jarreau joins Julia and David Koch at the Las Vegas Invitational.

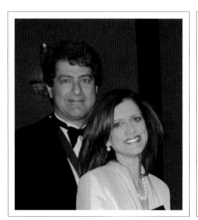
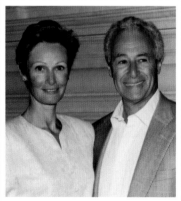

Leon and Debbie Black (left) and Pamela and Marty Wygod (right) have been among the PCF's leading supporters since its inception.

Johnny Mathis

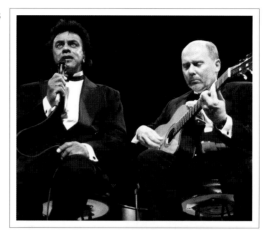

Sugar Ray Leonard
and Pete Sampras
with PCF Chairman
Mike Milken

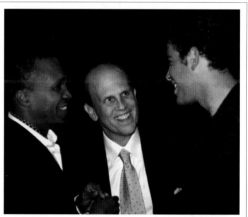

George Clooney and
Don Cheadle

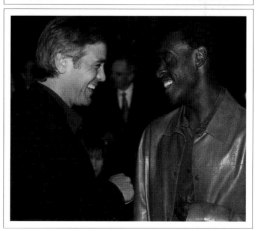

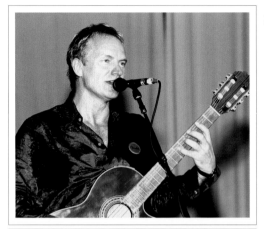

Sting

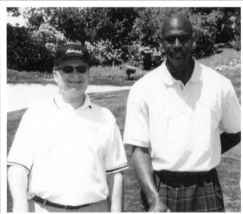

Tom Lee and
Michael Jordan

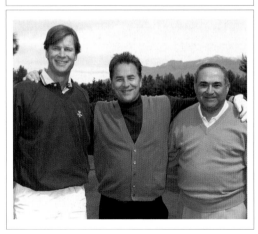

Ted Virtue,
Don Johnson and
Cano Ozgener

Wolfgang Reitzle,
(then actor, now
Governor)
Arnold
Schwarzenegger
and
Les Moonves

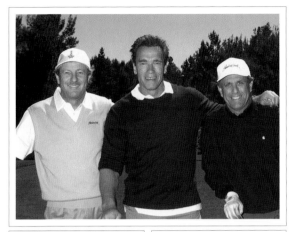

Will Smith and
Matt Damon

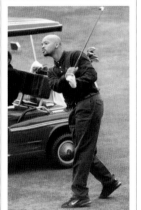
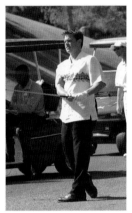

Robert Wagner
and
Jill St. John

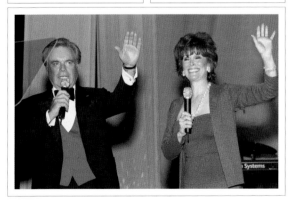

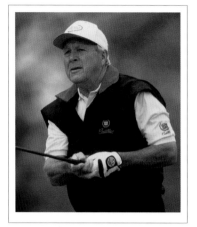
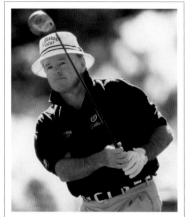

Golfing legend Arnold Palmer (left) and PGA Champions Tour star Jim Colbert, both prostate cancer survivors, were honored at the 1998 PCF New York Dinner. In conjunction with the PGA Champions Tour, the PCF has raised millions of dollars for prostate cancer research.

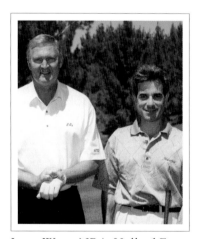
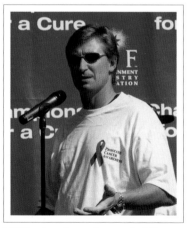

Jerry West, NBA Hall of Fame baseketball player (left) and Howard Scher, M.D., a PCF-supported researcher at Memorial Sloan-Kettering Cancer Center.

NHL hockey legend Wayne Gretzky has appeared at several PCF fund-raising events.

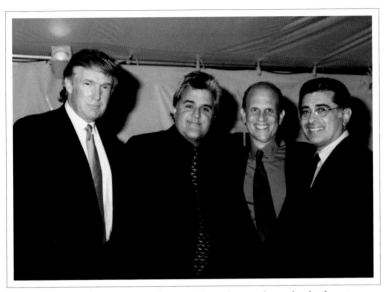

In early 1998, the Prostate Cancer Foundation launched what is now the Carl H. Lindner Pro-Am Invitational tennis tournament at Donald Trump's Mar-a-Lago Club in Palm Beach. Left to right: Donald Trump, Jay Leno, Mike Milken and Yahoo! Chairman Terry Semel.

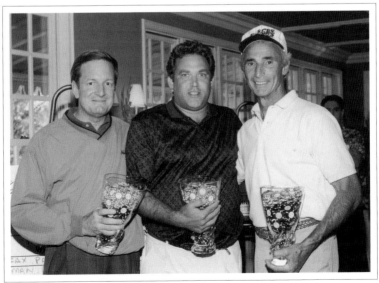

Businessman and investor Ronald Burkle (left), who has supported a wide range of PCF activities, joined Bruce Parker (center) and Sandy Koufax, Hall of Fame Dodgers' pitcher, at the Las Vegas Invitational.

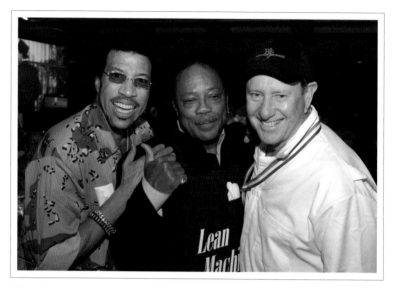

The Gourmet Games, a series of competitive food tastings, is a fund-raising event that shows business leaders, entertainers and athletes healthful alternatives to high-fat foods. Above, Lionel Richie, Quincy Jones and businessman Bill Tilley show off their team uniforms at the 2002 Los Angeles Gourmet Games. Below, cell phone pioneer Craig McCaw jokes with PCF Chairman Mike Milken at the Seattle Gourmet Games in 2003.

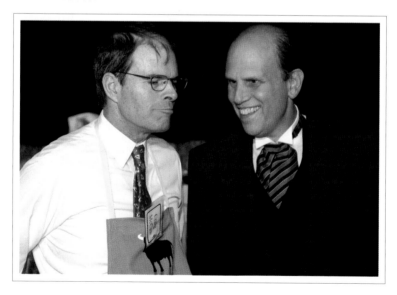

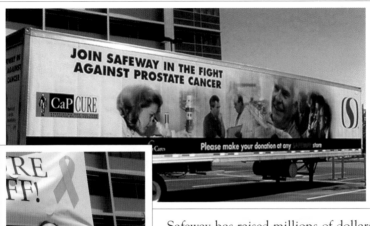

Safeway has raised millions of dollars for the PCF through corporate and employee-funded donations and from customers at check stands nationwide. Left, Safeway CEO and Chairman Steve Burd launches its annual prostate cancer campaign; above, the company promotes its corporate effort on its trucks.

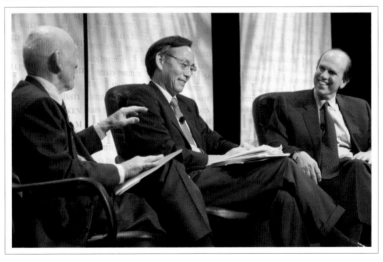

The Global Conferences of the Milken Institute, an economic think tank, have increasingly focused on medical research issues. Nobel laureates Paul Boyer and Steven Chu with panel moderator Mike Milken.

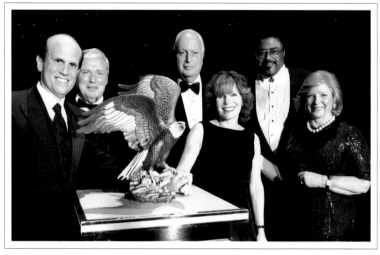

Mike and Lori Milken were honored for more than a quarter-century of support for medical research at the PCF's 2003 New York Dinner. From left: Mike Milken; NCI Director Andrew von Eschenbach, M.D.; PCF board member Mickey Tarnopol; Lori Milken; PCF board member Rosey Grier; and Lynne Tarnopol.

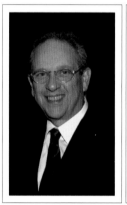 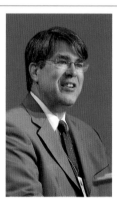 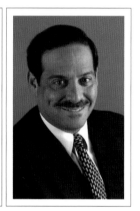

Stuart "Skip" Holden, M.D., PCF medical director.

Howard Soule, Ph.D., PCF chief science officer.

Leslie Michelson, PCF vice chairman and chief executive officer.

months since his prostate cancer diagnosis the previous spring, Torre had become a highly visible public spokesman for the PCF by appearing in public service announcements and participating actively in the Home Run Challenge (see Chapter 10). Steve Wynn delivered a moving tribute to the scientists searching for a cure and the contributors who support their work.

At the 2001 New York Dinner, just two months after the 9/11 attacks, producer David Foster led the entire ballroom in singing *God Bless America* to honor New York's heroes including, on the stage, members of the New York Fire Department. Also honored that evening were the Mack brothers – David, Bill, Fred and Earle – for their widespread philanthropy that includes, in addition to support of the Prostate Cancer Foundation, major gifts to the Long Island Jewish Health System, whose North Shore University Hospital was ranked the number-one hospital in the U.S. by the AARP.

Whoopi Goldberg returned to host the 10th anniversary dinner in 2003, an event that featured a version of Cher's Farewell Tour concert. Reporting on the performance in her newspaper column, Liz Smith said, "By the time she got to the [last number], the ballroom was on its feet." Mike and Lori Milken were honorees at the dinner, which raised more than $5 million for cancer research.

A personal commitment

The motivation of many contributors to be personally involved – to host fund-raisers or to participate actively in the medical research process year after year – often stems from personal experience. Prostate-cancer survivor David Koch (see Chapter 6) and his wife, Julia, have provided nearly $100 million to a wide range of endeavors. Koch and his family have established the David H. Koch Prostate Cancer Research Awards. These awards have enabled the PCF to provide more than $6 million to fund major research programs at The Johns Hopkins University, M.D. Anderson Cancer Center, and Memorial Sloan-Kettering Cancer

Center. But Koch has done far more than donate money. He has become deeply and personally involved in advancing the programs of the institutions he supports. He has participated actively in PCF Scientific Retreats; he meets with scientists and research physicians to better understand their needs and aspirations; and he confers regularly with biotechnology and pharmaceutical companies to discuss commercialization of work he has funded.

S. Ward Casscells, M.D., known to his friends as "Trip," is a distinguished cardiologist and professor of medicine at the University of Texas. Following a diagnosis of advanced prostate cancer that had invaded dozens of his bones, Casscells thought he was going to die within a matter of months. Then he consulted Dr. Christopher Logothetis, a prostate cancer expert at the M.D. Anderson Cancer Center. Vowing to "fix you up," Logothetis instituted an aggressive integrated treatment regimen of hormones and chemotherapy that was developed through research funded by the PCF. Dr. Casscells is so grateful that he joined the PCF board and agreed to tell his story in a direct-mail piece that the PCF uses to raise funds:

> "I could have easily been a statistic. But thanks to the Prostate Cancer Foundation and the scientists and research they support, I'm alive to tell you about it. I'm feeling good. And I look forward to seeing my young children graduate."

In many cases, despite the fact that prostate cancer physically affects men, it's also a wife, a mother or a sister who is profoundly affected. Longtime PCF supporter Lynda Resnick wrote:

> "Silver picture frames glisten on my table. Faces of the ones I love smile back at me. I see Grandpa, the kindest, most supportive and loving man I ever knew. He always was and still is my guardian angel. In my twenties, he was stolen away by prostate cancer.

> "Then there's the picture of Uncle Bob – my hero. Only six years my senior, he was more like a big brother. He treated me like a princess. At 50, he was stricken with prostate cancer. I

watched helplessly as he suffered and died. He left a loving wife and two teenage boys. As a wife, mother and sister, I know the men I love are at risk. The only way to deal with the threat is to fight back. And I am."

For Resnick, vice chairman of The Franklin Mint, fighting back has entailed much more than generous financial support – hosting a highly successful West Coast fund-raiser in her home, playing a leadership role on the board of directors and, along with her husband, Stewart, attending PCF events throughout the year.

When brothers Bruce and John Nordstrom and their sister, Anne Gittinger, lost their brother, James, to prostate cancer, they wanted to expand their philanthropy to help fight the disease. Along with Anne's husband, Wayne, they made a large personal commitment to the PCF, which expands on their family's corporate philanthropy that supports community development, education, the arts and health services through the Nordstrom stores.

Reaching a national audience

Andy Grove, chairman of Intel Corporation, focused his financial and intellectual capital on beating the disease when was diagnosed with prostate cancer in the mid-1990s. He joined the PCF board, contributed important business insights to the PCF Therapy Consortium, and told his personal story in a *Fortune* magazine cover article.

Grove's openness about his disease probably encouraged other public figures to talk about their prostate cancer diagnoses. Milken had been one of the first to go public in 1993. He felt that the simple act of announcing your diagnosis could save lives by generating news coverage that would be read by millions of men. That would create awareness and motivate many of them to see their doctors for a PSA test. Senator John Kerry, General Schwarzkopf, Rupert Murdoch, Joe Torre and dozens of other public figures followed Milken's example in making public announcements. For someone famous, it is as important a way of giving as writing a check.

For many years, Safeway Corporation had supported breast cancer research. In 2001, Safeway employees made a commitment to support prostate cancer research, contributing money and setting up checkout counter displays in thousands of stores so that customers nationwide could learn more and make donations (see Chapter 10).

Other charities established in the last decade have followed models similar to the one created by the PCF. After many years of continuing major support for the PCF, Charles Dolan, founder and chairman of Cablevision Systems Corporation, and his son, James, wanted to expand their philanthropy to support pancreatic cancer research. With the help of the PCF, the Dolans established the Lustgarten Foundation for Pancreatic Cancer Research in 1998, implementing many of the PCF's most innovative strategies, such as an annual scientific conference and fast-track grant applications. And like the PCF, Lustgarten has worked closely with the National Cancer Institute to ensure funding of a SPORE grant (see Chapter 5) in pancreatic cancer. Accelerate Brain Cancer Cure (ABC[2]), like the PCF, has established a fast-track award process that limits applications to five pages.

A Wynning hand

Over the past three decades, more than any other person, Steve Wynn has revitalized Las Vegas. Wynn's vision of building hotels on a grand scale that offered impeccable service, elegance and activities for families – in essence, an 'adult Disneyland' – was a radical departure from traditional Las Vegas and helped boost its struggling economy in the 1980s. The Bellagio, Mirage and Treasure Island were ambitious hotels that conveyed an image beyond their casinos, at once featuring a collection of some of the world's greatest paintings, fine restaurants and shops, and dazzling outdoor shows. Continuing this tradition, Wynn Resorts is building Wynn Las Vegas, scheduled to open in 2005 as the preeminent luxury hotel in the city. Wynn's devotion to his work and to numerous charities is matched by his wife's commitment. A leading education advocate in Nevada, Elaine Wynn joined the

Prostate Cancer Foundation board of directors in 1995. The Wynns established the Shadow Creek Golf Invitational to support the PCF. Shadow Creek built on the PCF tradition of inviting top entertainers, athletes and committed advocates for increased cancer research funding. (After the sale of Wynn's company to Kirk Kerkorian's MGM Grand, the Shadow Creek tradition continued with the support of Kerkorian, Bobby Baldwin and Terri Lanni.)

Investor Thomas H. Lee and art collector Ann Tenenbaum (now Mrs. Lee) were among the first to commit to the Shadow Creek tournament. (When Milken was diagnosed in 1993, Tenenbaum had urged him to consider the effect a positive attitude could have on the disease, and joined him at a meeting of the American Psychosocial Oncology Society.) Other major Shadow Creek supporters have included such business leaders as Herb Kohler, Scott McNealy, Kerry Packer, Len Riggio, Ed Rontell, Ted Virtue and Stanley Zax, who has been a member of the PCF board of directors since its founding. Over the years, guests have mingled with actors George Clooney, Kevin Costner, Matt Damon, Michael Douglas, Clint Eastwood, Jack Nicholson, Will Smith, Sylvester Stallone and (then actor, now California Governor) Arnold Schwarzenegger, as well as with such great athletes as Julius Erving, Wayne Gretzky, Hale Irwin, Michael Jordan, Sandy Koufax, Sugar Ray Leonard, Greg Norman, Pete Sampras, and Jerry West. Entertainers at Shadow Creek have included Paul Anka, Celine Dion, Kenny G, Vince Gill, Amy Grant, Josh Groban, Kenny Loggins and Lionel Richie.

Attending his first Shadow Creek event following his naming as the PCF's vice chairman and chief executive officer in 2002, Leslie Michelson was struck by the celebrity of the assembled guests.

> *"If you think about it, ten years ago, prostate cancer was virtually unknown and there was no Prostate Cancer Foundation. Look what's happened in a decade. Not only have we made great strides in medical science, but we've also been able*

to attract many of the world's top business leaders and enter-
tainment figures to help our cause. And look at the sports stars
– Gretzky, Jordan, Leonard, Sampras and the others. They're
the absolute best in their fields. It's quite impressive."

Keeping up with Tiger

Many of the PCF's major supporters have hosted events infused
with their own personalities. One of the earliest was Marvin
Shanken, the publisher of *Wine Spectator* magazine, who began
hosting an annual *A Night to Remember* dinner. The evening's
highlight is an extraordinary auction that includes such donated
items as exclusive luxury vacations, golfing packages, rare wines,
and Super Bowl tickets.

In early 1998, the PCF launched what was to become the Carl H.
Lindner Pro-Am Invitational tennis tournament at Donald
Trump's Mar-a-Lago Club in Palm Beach. Current and retired
tennis stars like Jimmy Connors, Chris Evert Lloyd, Mats Wilander
and Andrea Jaeger are paired with amateurs for the round-robin
tournament to raise money for prostate cancer research. Lindner,
one of America's leading philanthropists and the owner of the
Cincinnati Reds, has hosted a variety of events in support of the
PCF's Home Run Challenge (HRC). Other contributors through
the HRC have included investor Cliff Robbins and restaurant-
chain owner Jamie Coulter (see Chapter 10).

At the end of 1998, philanthropists R. D. and Joan Dale Hubbard
hosted the first Benefit at BIGHORN at one of the premier golf
courses in the West. The Hubbards joined with Senior Tour golfer
Jim Colbert launching the golf tournament and a country-western
dinner where the chili was spicy and the dress strictly sequins and
boots. Guests golfed with many of the stars from the PGA
Champions Tour, including such legends as Colbert, Hale Irwin
and Lee Trevino. Earl Woods, father of Tiger Woods and a
prostate-cancer survivor, even gave some BIGHORN guests a golf
lesson, apparently with mixed results. *"Now I shoot the same score*
as Tiger," joked one celebrity duffer, *"Except that I do it in nine holes*
and he does it in 18."

A golfing legend from an earlier era, Arnold Palmer, lends his name and involvement to Arnie's Army Battles Prostate Cancer, which raises funds and generates public awareness. The PCF and the Professional Golfers Association have enlisted more than 1,500 golf courses across America to sponsor closest-to-the-pin contests on par-3 holes. Tee markers, banners, pin flags and other materials carry the message encouraging golfers to join Arnie's Army and donate money to defeat prostate cancer.

In 2002, Montana businessman Dennis Washington and his wife, Phyllis, joined with Charles Pasarell Jr. and Raymond J. Moore of PM Sports Management to introduce the Indian Wells (California) Tennis Invitational, a pro/am doubles tournament held in conjunction with the Pacific Life Tennis Open. In contrast to the western flavor of the Benefit at BIGHORN, the Indian Wells event features an elegant dinner where guests arrive dressed all in white. Players include two dozen current and former top-ranked professionals including Tracy Austin, John Lloyd, Eddie Dibbs and Cliff Drysdale, as well as former Canadian teenage-ranked tennis player, Matthew Perry, star of Friends, and NHL Hall of Famer Wayne Gretzky with his actress wife, Janet Jones.

Gourmet Games

The PCF has been a leader in funding medical research projects exploring the role of nutrition (see Chapter 11). The organization quickly learned that one way to help people realize the benefits of a healthier diet was to "let them taste it for themselves." The PCF often serves event guests what they think are traditional high-fat foods like spaghetti Bolognese, Reuben sandwiches and chocolate pudding. In fact, they are low-fat meals made with healthy ingredients, often soy-based products cleverly disguised to have the same look, aroma and taste as the original.

Many of these recipes are featured in *The Taste for Living Cookbook*, which Milken co-authored with chef Beth Ginsberg. Few people can differentiate between the low-fat and the more-traditional high-calorie versions they're used to eating. The taste tests have worked at dinner parties, in the U.S. Senate dining room and perhaps most convincingly, at a party for a group of noisy, young kids at Lake Tahoe.

The PCF was determined to link its message about healthy eating and lifestyles with a fund-raising opportunity. The Gourmet Games was the perfect opportunity. Inaugurated with the support of California businessmen Bill Tilley, Marc Nathanson, Stewart Resnick and Bobby Kotick, the Gourmet Games feature an entertaining set of food-and-wine tasting and trivia competitions, pitting teams of business leaders, athletes, entertainers and physicians against each other. Dressed in team regalia and with team names like The *Sip*ranos, the Milken Honeys, the Galloping Gourmets and the Dirty Dozen, such celebrities as Warren Beatty, Quincy Jones, Sidney Poitier, Matthew McConnaughey and many others take turns tasting red and white wines, soups, salads, entrées and desserts. Competing alongside teammates such as Hilton president and CEO Stephen Bollenbach, Heritage Provider Network CEO Richard Merkin, M.D., and Platinum Equity Chairman Tom Gores, teams build up points by trying to discern which foods are lowest in fat and which wines come from which regions of the world, or by getting the correct answers to difficult trivia quizzes.

Not all PCF contributions have come from wealthy donors. The importance of the organization's cause has brought touching support from unexpected sources. Each spring, hundreds of current and former winners of the Milken Family Foundation's National Education Award gather in Los Angeles for an education conference and awards dinner. Art Reisman, a 1989 Milken Educator honoree from Illinois, remembers an evening in 1995:

"It was a spontaneous thing just before the awards dinner. The Illinois delegation wanted to express its appreciation to the Milken Family Foundation for everything it had done, and one of us had heard about the Prostate Cancer Foundation, which was just getting started at the time. Our delegation collected more than $1,000, put it in an envelope and decided we would donate it to the PCF. Then we asked Mike Milken to stop in at our delegation meeting, which of course he did, bringing his mother with him. We presented Mike with the envelope – it was all very emotional. Mike was in tears. It was very surprising and moving for everyone."

As it enters its second decade, the PCF is a more mature organization whose strategies are evolving. The PCF is now focused on continuing to build public awareness and on broadening the base of its fund-raising activities. Several organizations are helping in these efforts by contributing pro-bono services and support that have already exceeded $1 million in value. Among these organizations are TBWA\Chiat\Day, the international advertising agency; Porter Novelli, one of the world's largest public relations organizations; Arnold & Porter and FoxKiser, two distinguished Washington-based law firms; and Burns McClellan, a prominent biotechnology public relations company.

Keeping Dad in the Game

Going to a baseball game with your father or grandfather is a great American tradition, a rite of passage that generations of boys and girls now grown older won't soon forget – clinging tightly to a grownup's hand as they entered a larger-than-life stadium for the first time, cheering the home team until they were hoarse, and eating some peanuts and Cracker Jack™. But above all, baseball is about the excitement of that singular moment – the crack of the bat as legendary players like Willie Mays, Mickey Mantle or Barry Bonds smash towering home runs.

With its cherished place in the heart of America, what better setting than a baseball park to raise awareness about prostate cancer – a disease that strikes dads and granddads everywhere – and to raise money to fund research? And what more appropriate time than Father's Day? In 1995, Mike Milken and Rosey Grier began planning what would become the Prostate Cancer Foundation's Home Run Challenge (HRC).

Since 1998, the program has grown considerably under the direction of Dave Perron, who was formerly with the Oakland Athletics. By 2003, the Home Run Challenge had become a massive awareness program promoted in nationally broadcast radio and television public service announcements, dozens of on-air mentions during games, and ceremonies at all 30 Major League Baseball ballparks. No other program has done more to bring the facts about prostate cancer to American men and their families.

It was introduced as "The Father's Day Campaign" in 1996. The Kansas City Royals, San Francisco Giants, Atlanta Braves and

Anaheim Angels each donated thousands of tickets that the PCF distributed to prostate cancer survivors. In 1997, the Home Run Challenge grew to include all Major League Baseball teams. Individual fans and businesses around the world pledged anywhere from $1 to $10,000 for each home run hit in each of 60 pre-selected games during the week of Father's Day. Scores of sluggers like Jason Giambi, Tim Salmon, Roberto Alomar, Jeff Bagwell, Jim Thome and Eric Karros have hit some 800 home runs during HRC games.

Publicity for the HRC takes a chilling statistic about prostate cancer and relates it to baseball:

> *"If baseball were played around the clock every day of the year, 54 American men would be diagnosed with prostate cancer during each game – one for every out – and nine would die from the disease – one every inning."*

Blue everywhere

The Home Run Challenge involves more than players. Through its partnership with Major League Baseball, the PCF enlists managers, umpires, groundskeepers, trainers and owners to "Keep Dad in the Game." A Home Run Challenge game is a festive event awash in a sea of baby blue (the color of the prostate cancer ribbon). Players wear blue prostate cancer pins, wristbands, blue eye glare and temporary tattoos. Pre-game ceremonies often recognize local ballplayers, donors, celebrities and prostate cancer survivors. In many stadiums, groundskeepers put their artistic skills to work painting the blue ribbon on the grass along the foul lines.

Major League stars like Alex Rodriguez, Mike Sweeney, Chipper Jones, Shawn Green and Carlos Delgado have conducted broadcast interviews wearing blue eye glare and pointing out its significance as they asked for pledges. Players like Ken Griffey Jr., Derek Jeter and Sammy Sosa and managers like Joe Torre and Dusty Baker (both prostate cancer survivors) are featured by such official HRC

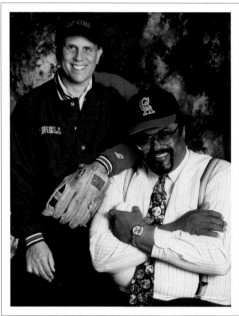

Mike Milken and Rosey Grier, former NFL Pro Bowl star and PCF board member, developed an idea to promote awareness of prostate cancer with Major League Baseball. Since 1996, the PCF Home Run Challenge has raised nearly $20 million.

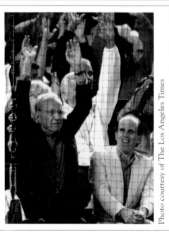

Photo courtesy of The Los Angeles Times

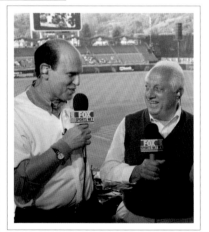

The Prostate Cancer Foundation's Home Run Challenge has grown into a massive awareness and fund-raising program for prostate cancer research promoted in conjunction with Major League Baseball (MLB), radio and television stations and all 30 MLB teams. News Corp. Chairman Rupert Murdoch (left), former owner of the Los Angeles Dodgers, does 'The Wave' as Mike Milken looks on. Hall of Fame Dodgers Manager Tommy Lasorda (right) travels across the country every year and appears at games and on countless television and radio programs to raise awareness about prostate cancer.

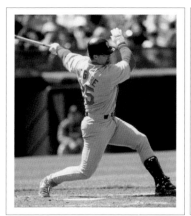

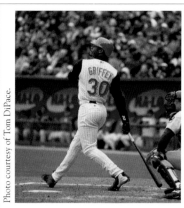

Photo courtesy of Tom DiPace.

Future Hall of Fame slugger Mark McGwire hit six home runs in Home Run Challenge games.

Ken Griffey Jr. is a featured PCF star. Each home run hit during 60 selected games in the week before Father's Day raises money for prostate cancer research.

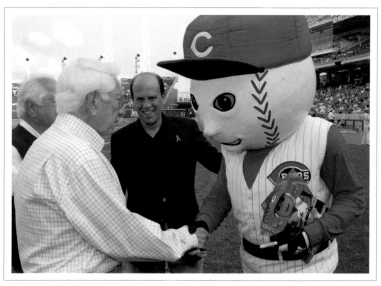

Cincinnati Reds Owner Carl Lindner (left) is a major supporter of the Prostate Cancer Foundation's Home Run Challenge.

media sponsors as FOX Networks, Time Warner, Turner Broadcasting and Yahoo! in public service announcements. In one announcement, Yankees manager Torre says: *"We've kept quiet about this disease for too long. Prostate cancer poses a serious risk – especially to men over 40. It's time we did something about it."* Torre has also appeared on such national broadcasts as *The Charlie Rose Show* in connection with the HRC.

In addition to broadcasting many of the games on his Fox Sports unit, News Corporation Chairman and former L.A. Dodgers owner Rupert Murdoch has been one of the largest contributors to the Home Run Challenge. Among many other top HRC supporters are team owners and partners like Carl Lindner (Cincinnati Reds), Steve Geppi (Baltimore Orioles), and Peter Magowan (San Francisco Giants); and such business leaders as Bob Barth, Leon Black, Ron Burkle, Charles Dolan, Mel Karmazin, Art Kern, Terry Semel, Ed Snider and Eddie Trump. Other owners and partners including the New York Mets' Fred Wilpon, the Boston Red Sox's John Henry and Larry Lucchino, the Atlanta Braves' former owner Ted Turner, the Yankees' George Steinbrenner, the Seattle Mariners' Wayne Perry, and the Colorado Rockies' Jerry McMorris have hosted the PCF at their stadiums.

The PCF's Home Run Challenge team crisscrosses the country attending as many as three games per day when they can catch an afternoon contest and the beginning of a night game on the East Coast and then fly west for a later night game. The group often brings along former All-Stars, such as Terry Steinbach, and Hall of Fame members including Reggie Jackson, Ernie Banks, Dennis Eckersley, and former Dodgers manager Tommy Lasorda. One of baseball's greatest ambassadors, Lasorda travels tirelessly for the HRC year after year, flying thousands of miles to speak with fans, promote the need for men to get PSA tests, and urge people to support the Prostate Cancer Foundation. Speaking at a 2003 event with Milken nearby, Lasorda said:

"I believe this as much as I believe I'm standing here. If anybody, anybody, is going to find a cure for prostate cancer, it's that fellow – Mike Milken – right over there. He's given up time, money and energy to do this, and I'm so happy and proud just to go alongside of him so that one day we'll have a cure for this destructive disease."

Special moments

The Home Run Challenge has also included a "bonus game" that isn't quite Major League, but is major fun – the Congressional baseball game in suburban Washington that matches Democratic and Republican lawmakers in a good-natured contest for charity.

There have also been emotional moments. In 2001, the Philadelphia Phillies' Brian Hunter stood at home plate with his father, a prostate cancer survivor, for a pre-game presentation. Oakland A's pitcher Gil Heredia presented his father, also a prostate cancer survivor, with a blue wristband at the start of a game. And the entire Minnesota Twins team wore initialed blue wristbands to honor the memory of a teammate's father who died on the morning of Father's Day.

Each year, in June, the Safeway Corporation raises millions of dollars for prostate cancer research with its own funding drive and awareness campaign. Through the leadership of Chairman and CEO Steve Burd, Safeway encourages customers to contribute to prostate cancer research with point-of-purchase promotions at thousands of checkout stands in 1,700 North American stores. The company's franchises include Safeway, Vons, Pavilions, Carrs, Randalls, Tom Thumb, Dominick's, and Genuardi's – all of which feature in-store promotions and blue-ribbon tear-off sheets. Safeway has also promoted involvement with large signs on the sides of trucks. These materials raise awareness by urging the public to "join Safeway in the fight against prostate cancer."

Safeway also makes an annual corporate and employee-funded donation to the PCF. And the company raises funds for the PCF at an annual softball game pitting Safeway executives against the Nabisco Traveling All-Star team, which includes such former Major League Baseball stars as Steve Carlton, Ron Cey and Steve Garvey. Another corporate sponsor, AriZona Beverage Co, has installed aisle displays at all Safeway stores and designated a portion of each sale to benefit the PCF. Finally, in what has become a tradition, Lasorda and PCF executives visit Safeway stores each year during the Home Run Challenge to bag groceries and help customers take the bags to their cars.

Several other corporations have joined the PCF's team during the Home Run Challenge. H.J. Heinz, in conjunction with Safeway, Kroger and other stores, has featured in-store promotions and incentives for shoppers to make contributions to prostate cancer research. Corporate executives such as Lone Star Steakhouse's CEO Jamie Coulter, have traveled the country to help draw attention to the Home Run Challenge mission, and Men's Health magazine, Macy's, and Yahoo! have also participated.

Over the years, the HRC has featured many special moments, from Mark McGwire's and Sammy Sosa's assault on Roger Maris' 37-year-old home run record in 1998, to Roger Clemens' attempts to notch his 300th career win, to the no-hitter thrown against the New York Yankees in 2003 by six Houston Astros pitchers. Most exciting of all, however, is the nearly $20 million the Home Run Challenge has brought in for prostate cancer research.

Prevention Beats Treatment

*E*rnst Wynder, M.D. had always been a maverick, a man ahead of his time. The German-born physician and researcher, who died in 1999, was credited with co-authoring the first study definitively linking lung cancer and smoking in 1950 – a full 14 years before the U.S. Surgeon General. Continuing his pioneering work, he began studying the relationship between lifestyle and cancer, only to be frustrated by the lack of interest and funding. In 1969, he left the prestigious Memorial Sloan-Kettering Cancer Center in New York to form the American Health Foundation, where he was free to delve into the role that smoking, diet and alcohol played in raising cancer risks.

Among those who recognized Wynder's research was the Milken Family Foundation, which gave him a Cancer Research Award in 1990. Yet, nearly 50 years after he sounded the alarm on smoking, and 25 years after warning that diet could affect disease, many researchers doubted his nutrition research. As Milken recalled:

"We now know that about 70 percent of healthcare spending in America – $1 trillion – is spent on lifestyle-related diseases. Yet for quite a while, few medical researchers studied or advocated prevention strategies. The public has responded much more quickly, especially in recognizing the benefits of nutrition. You see it, for example, in the explosion of soy products. The fact is, there are substantially different death rates in countries with different diets. And in many cases, when people from other countries with lower death rates for certain diseases come to America, within one generation they become more susceptible to the same diseases."

Building on growing interest in how a healthy lifestyle and diet could affect cancer, the PCF's second Scientific Retreat at Santa Barbara in 1994 featured a contentious panel discussion on nutrition. For some researchers, this was the first time they had actually seen hard data on nutrition research.

"We presented some ideas about developing a soy-based formula for prostate cancer patients, and it turned into more of a debate about the efficacy of nutrition research," remembers David Heber, M.D., Ph.D., now director of the UCLA Center for Human Nutrition.

Following the Retreat debate, there were increased calls for more scientific nutritional research. With substantial input from the PCF, the National Institutes of Health (NIH) responded by including nutrition research funding in its prostate cancer strategic plan.

"Since that first year," Heber says, *"the nutrition sessions have become a staple of the Retreat, and the data presented have become more substantial. There's a tremendous amount of interest, both from researchers and patients."*

Better than the salad bar

One of the researchers at the PCF Retreat was William Nelson, M.D., a Johns Hopkins University researcher who studies how diet affects prostate cancer.

"The PCF takes an approach that I didn't even dare to think about – whether you can change the way people eat on a larger scale and change how they view their health," Nelson says. *"I'm in the lab trying to divine which foods to avoid and which can be helpful, and then get that information out. That's as far as I thought we could take it. The PCF sees things on a grander scale. With that same data, they believed that we could actively steer people toward a better diet if we could make it more attractive to the palate. In other words, don't just spend every day foraging around the salad bar, but make an entire cuisine that's healthy. It's been fabulous to watch."*

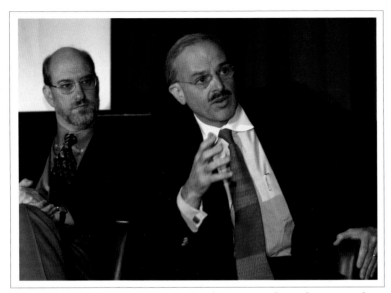

The PCF has been a pioneer in funding research to determine how nutrition affects cancer and other serious diseases. David Heber, M.D., Ph.D., (right), director of the UCLA Center for Human Nutrition, is joined at the 2003 Scientific Retreat by Eric Klein, M.D., section head of urologic oncology at The Cleveland Clinic.

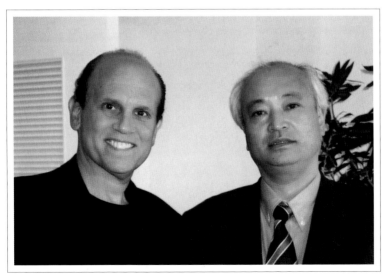

The PCF has funded international studies on the effect of nutrition, including a joint project between UCLA researchers and Munekado Kojima, M.D., director of the Nagoya Urology Hospital in Japan.

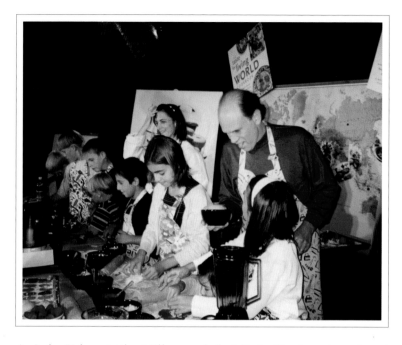

At Lake Tahoe, Mike Milken and chef Beth Ginsberg introduced healthful *Taste for Living* cookbook recipes to a tough audience – kids.

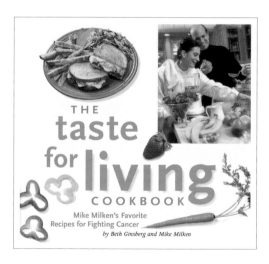

As a result of his advanced prostate cancer diagnosis, Milken radically restructured his diet so he could enjoy his favorite dishes with low-fat, soy-based ingredients in place of traditionally high-fat foods. He and Beth Ginsberg co-authored a best-selling cookbook.

What Nelson and others have been watching is the acceleration of the PCF's leadership in the nutrition field, both by funding scientific research and by raising public awareness. While studies are not yet conclusive, evidence from clinical trials at UCLA, Memorial Sloan-Kettering Cancer Center and the Preventive Medicine Research Institute suggests that a low-fat, high-fiber diet may be helpful.

The UCLA Center for Human Nutrition, headed by Dr. Heber, is one of the nation's leading nutrition research centers. He cites several studies among a greatly expanded body of scientific nutritional knowledge:

- Heber's lab has shown that increased levels of lycopene (abundant in cooked tomatoes) in the blood and a reduction in polyunsaturated fats relate to reduced PSA levels in some men. There are also indications from studies in animals that green tea may inhibit the spread of prostate cancer. Another study provides a biological rationale for the association of obesity and prostate cancer – when overweight men lose weight, their blood has less of the inflammatory substances that are believed to promote prostate cancer.

- Dr. Nelson at Johns Hopkins has determined that prostate cancer cells acquire a vulnerability to gene-damaging carcinogens in red meat, and that substances found in vegetables such as broccoli may protect against carcinogens and genetic damage.

- The late William Fair, M.D., former chief of urology at the Memorial Sloan-Kettering Cancer Center, showed conclusively that human tumors implanted in animals grew more slowly when the animals were fed a diet comprising 20 percent fat compared to a diet with 40 percent fat. (The diets of many Americans are closer to 40 percent fat.) His research suggested that dietary intervention may be able to slow the progression of prostate cancer so that men would ultimately die decades later from something else.

- A study by Leonard Marks, M.D., a UCLA clinical urologist, in conjunction with Munekado Kojima, M.D., director of the Nagoya Urology Hospital in Japan, Dr. Heber and others, examined the diets and prostate tissue of Japanese men and men of Japanese ancestry born in the U.S. Milken later met with Dr. Kojima during a trip to Japan and discussed the study's findings with him. The study concluded that the Japanese urban diet had changed so much that there were only minor differences from the diets of Japanese-Americans living in California. The introduction of Western foods in Japan has increased the incidence of obesity there from five to 20 percent in just 20 years. So it is really the Japanese rural diet of 20 years ago that explains why prostate cancer rates are as much as ten times higher among American men than Japanese men. (Commenting on this finding, PCF board member Andy Grove proposed continued nutritional studies: *"Someone could get a Nobel Prize if they could figure out how to reduce the U.S. death rate by 90 percent down to the Japanese level."*)

In 1996, the PCF sponsored its first Nutritional Summit in Santa Monica, California to promote study of the effect of diet on the progression or recurrence of prostate cancer. At the time, the PCF awarded $750,000 to nutritional research efforts in New York, San Francisco and Los Angeles. The PCF eventually formed its own Nutrition Project, similar to its Therapy Consortium, bringing together researchers to exchange findings and plan future studies.

In 1997, the PCF published a monograph, Nutrition & Prostate Cancer, featuring the work of Dr. Heber; Dr. Fair; Dean Ornish, M.D., president and director of the Preventive Medicine Research Institute; and Dr. Wynder, the dean of nutrition researchers. The report, citing clinical trials underway at the Memorial Sloan-Kettering Cancer Center and at UCLA, detailed dietary components that may prevent the onset or recurrence of prostate cancer. The monograph focused on the effects of diet in conjunction with conventional treatments, especially hormone ablation, calorie restriction, fat intake, and the use of vitamin E, vitamin D and calcium.

Cooking for health

By 2004, the Prostate Cancer Foundation had funded more than
$4 million in Nutrition Project research and was also making
strong advances in building public awareness. In 1998, after more
than three years of testing and research, the PCF published *The
Taste for Living Cookbook: Mike Milken's Favorite Recipes for Fighting
Cancer*, combining nutritional guidelines with tasty, thoroughly
tested, easy-to-prepare recipes. This first cookbook emerged from
Milken's frustration with his fruit-and-steamed-vegetable diet
(see Chapter 4). Searching for a way to eat his favorite foods
without endangering his health, he hired Beth Ginsberg, a Los
Angeles chef with a reputation for healthful cooking. Ginsberg
worked with nutritionists to develop low-fat, soy-based versions of
such traditionally high-fat foods as puddings, cakes, sauce-laden
pastas, cheese-based dishes and much more. Distributed by Time-
Life Books, *Taste for Living* became a bestseller, buoyed by a cover
feature in *Newsweek* and by several national television appearances of Milken and Ginsberg.

The day after Milken's appearance with Barbara Walters, the
cookbook was the fourth-best-selling book on Amazon.com. He
also discussed nutrition on *The Charlie Rose Show* and *Access
Hollywood*, among others, and appeared with model Cindy
Crawford on *Larry King Live* to discuss healthy eating. The
resulting publicity not only helped sell cookbooks; it also encouraged people to think about what they ate and to get involved in
debates about such food-related matters as school lunches and
airline meals.

The cookbook and the PCF's research supported each other.
Recipes were based on the results of PCF-supported clinical trials.
At the same time, proceeds from the cookbooks were being
returned to the PCF to support additional prostate cancer and
nutrition research. The cookbooks translated clinical research
results into practical applications for people living with cancer.
Readers could find cancer-fighting meals created with low-fat or

soy-based ingredients – spaghetti Bolognese, quiche Lorraine and egg rolls – that didn't taste like they were created in a laboratory. And they could learn not only cooking techniques, but *why* certain ingredients were helpful to their health.

Other researchers are increasingly documenting the effects of poor diets on prostate cancer and other diseases, issues that the PCF began raising a decade ago. About 65 percent of Americans are now overweight or obese, and a *New England Journal of Medicine* study released in 2003 demonstrated that obesity may account for 14 percent of all cancer deaths among men, and 20 percent of cancer deaths among women. The result is 90,000 deaths every year. At the Dana Farber Cancer Institute, researcher Robert Mayer, M.D., reports that the effects of obesity make cancer harder to diagnose, more difficult to operate on, tougher to plan radiation therapy for, and less susceptible to chemotherapy.

Increasing obesity rates threaten more than just growing numbers of prostate and other cancer cases. Obesity has been identified as a precursor to heart disease, diabetes and a variety of other serious diseases. Americans now suffer from a record 17 million cases of diabetes, which not only causes devastating human suffering, but also drains the economy of at least $132 billion every year.

Fortunately, there is greater recognition of and respect for nutrition research than there was at the PCF's 1994 Scientific Retreat. The NIH continues to make nutrition research part of its funding, and the National Cancer Institute has included nutrition in recent studies on molecular markers in prostate cancer. At a recent meeting of C-Change, NCI Director Andrew von Eschenbach noted that obesity is a matter of not just too many calories, but poor-quality calories with too few fruits and vegetables and too much fat and hidden sugar and starches.

"It's remarkable to see the changes triggered in people, including those diagnosed with prostate cancer, who've changed their diets," adds Dr. Heber. "They've lost weight, increased their fitness levels, improved their quality of life and taken control of their disease. And they may have positively affected the biology of their prostate cancer. It may be several years before we have the final answer, but the PCF has changed the way we study nutrition."

Progress

*T*hroughout its first decade, the Prostate Cancer Foundation took a portfolio approach in funding early-stage innovative projects with the potential for breakthroughs against many diseases, not just prostate cancer. This is not unlike the business approach of venture capital firms, which invest in a diversified portfolio of companies, recognizing the high risk, but expecting that at least a few of them will be very successful in developing products that have broad applications.

The presence on the PCF board of directors of such innovators as Intel Chairman Andrew Grove and researcher/venture capitalist James Blair has helped integrate successful business principles from high-tech industries with good research ideas. As a result, the PCF has funded a series of significant studies that are helping to accelerate transfer of therapies from laboratories to doctors' offices. Obviously, some of these studies will be more successful than others. That's the nature of scientific investigation in any field. While some studies may turn out to be inconclusive, others will contribute to important breakthroughs. This chapter summarizes a few of the more promising steps by PCF supported researchers in a rough chronological sequence.

"We gotta cure this baby"

Jonathan Simons, M.D., then at Johns Hopkins University, used a 1995 PCF grant to develop an anti-prostate cancer vaccine, GVAX, which is currently undergoing clinical trials sponsored by the biotechnology company Cell Genesys. The vaccine contains a prostate-tumor-cell preparation that has been genetically engineered to express the protein GMCSF, which stimulates the patient's immune system to respond against the proteins unique to prostate cancer.

Now the head of the Winship Cancer Institute of Emory University in Atlanta, Simons and his colleague, Leland Chung, Ph.D., received a $10-million grant from the U.S. Department of Defense Prostate Cancer Research Program in 2003 for a "Manhattan Project" to address the problem of prostate cancer on several fronts (see Chapters 4 and 5). They are coordinating a massive program involving researchers at 13 universities in eight states. Among the participants are ten scientists and physicians, previously funded by the PCF, who have 150 years of funded investigator experience. Intel's Grove helped inspire the project, now called "A Synergy Consortium Targeting New Therapeutics for Lethal Phenotypes of Prostate Cancer."

This "Manhattan Project" is the first U.S. cancer research grant that uses web-based videoconferencing for daily and weekly research meetings as well as project management. The network creates "VCAPs" – Virtual Corridors of Adjacent Programs – a method of collaboration that allows the investigators to work as if they were just a hallway's walk away. Pointing to the advantages of this collaborative system, Simons quotes the original Manhattan Project head, J. Robert Oppenheimer, who led the wartime development of the atomic bomb and said (in 1944), "None of us is as smart as all of us." Dr. Chung concurs that multiple institutions will make faster progress against prostate cancer by synergistic collaboration. And he is dedicated to the success of the project, telling an early planning meeting, *"We gotta cure this baby."*

Vaccines-plus

Although GVAX shows promise, sometimes vaccines alone aren't enough.

In 1999, a PCF award went to James Allison, Ph.D., a molecular and cell biologist who is a professor of immunology at the University of California at Berkeley. Allison discovered an antibody that helps new vaccines work more effectively against prostate cancer cells. He is collaborating with Eric Small, M.D., at the University of California at San Francisco. Recognizing the market potential, the PCF worked with Allison and executives at the biotechnology firm Medarex to generate a plan to develop the drug for prostate cancer.

Allison's contribution is a monoclonal antibody to a molecule known as CTLA-4. In rodent models, he showed that antibodies to CTLA-4 enhanced immune responses to a level that could eradicate cancer even when given with weak vaccines. Based on these findings, clinical evaluations of the GVAX prostate cancer vaccine with Allison's monoclonal antibody are planned.

> "Cancer vaccines in general have not yet had a significant impact on the disease," says PCF Chief Science Officer Howard Soule. "Adding an adjuvant or supplementary treatment, however, has demonstrated great potential based on the pre-clinical trials. We've seen vaccines that previously had very little result all of a sudden cure rodents of their cancer. This is an area we're very excited about."

Anti-angiogenesis

A cancerous tumor needs its own blood supply to grow and spread throughout the body. The process of generating new blood vessels is called angiogenesis. Judah Folkman, M.D., at Children's Hospital Boston, first showed how this process worked. Folkman then pioneered the concept of anti-angiogenesis by searching for an agent to inhibit blood vessel formation at the site of tumors. It was thought that anti-angiogenesis would result in shrinking or eliminating tumors. The effects of Folkman's work – funded for five years by the PCF – have influenced not only prostate cancer research, but nearly every branch of oncology. Dozens of compounds have been discovered that inhibit angiogenesis. Today, the National Cancer Institute is sponsoring ongoing clinical trials of anti-angiogenesis drugs.

Early in 2004, the Food and Drug Administration (FDA) approved Genentech's Avastin, an anti-angiogenesis drug, for use in treating advanced colon cancer. Further trials of Avastin as a treatment for recurrent prostate cancer are expected. Illustrating the growth potential for companies that commit to developing drugs and treatments for cancer and other serious diseases, the price of Genentech stock soared on the day of the FDA announcement. In fact, the market capitalization of Genentech tripled – adding some $40 billion of value – in the ten months after it became apparent that Avastin was likely to be approved.

Surrogate markers

It can take as long as a decade to learn the effect of an experimental prostate cancer drug in men who receive it in controlled clinical trials. Traditionally, the only sure measure of effectiveness is to see how many men in each group died. Surrogate markers are indirect but accurate indicators that can predict what the future holds for a particular patient. "Surrogate" means that the indicator, or "marker," is a substitute for death or serious disease as the outcome of a clinical trial. For example, a high cholesterol reading increases the likelihood of future heart disease. If a new drug reduces cholesterol, doctors have more confidence that it will reduce the risk of heart attacks without having to wait a decade for mortality data. But it is difficult to establish these medical road signs with a precision acceptable to the FDA.

Harvard radiation oncologist Anthony D'Amico, M.D., Ph.D., with PCF funding, has shown that a doubling of the PSA score in three months or less is a strong predictor of when death will come for those who were treated by radiation therapy or surgery for primary prostate cancer. This surrogate marker may be crucial in qualifying drug candidates for accelerated FDA approval. Specifically, if a researcher can demonstrate that a drug reduces PSA scores in appropriate patients, that drug could be approved by the FDA in as little as one-third the usual time even before there is direct statistical proof of lives saved. For his pioneering work on

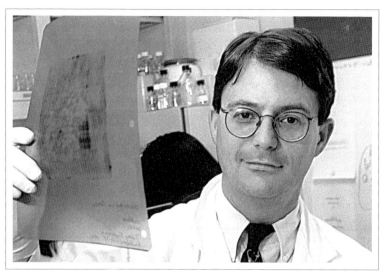

Jonathan Simons, M.D., was a young researcher at Johns Hopkins University when he received his first Prostate Cancer Foundation research award in 1995. Simons is now the director of the Winship Cancer Institute at Emory University, where he leads a 13-institution prostate cancer research consortium under a $10 million Defense Department grant.

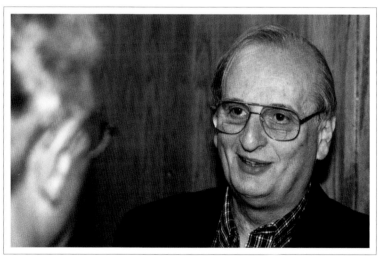

Judah Folkman, M.D., at Children's Hospital Medical Center in Boston, pioneered the concept of anti-angiogenesis to inhibit blood vessel formation at the site of tumors. His work – funded for five years by the PCF – has influenced not only prostate cancer research, but nearly every branch of oncology.

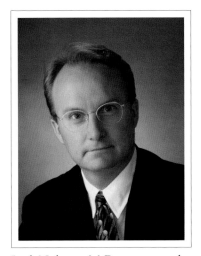

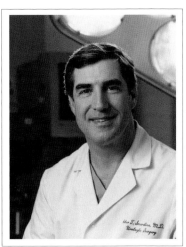

Joel Nelson, M.D., now at the University of Pittsburgh, led a PCF-supported research team that demonstrated that a cardiovascular drug, Atrasentan, alters the growth of prostate cancer metastasized to bone.

Peter Scardino, M.D., chairman of the Department of Urology at Memorial Sloan-Kettering Cancer Center, has received PCF awards for studies of surgical outcomes as a way to better predict the risk of prostate cancer recurrence.

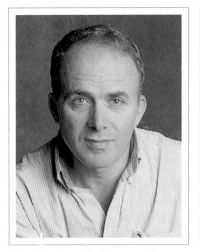

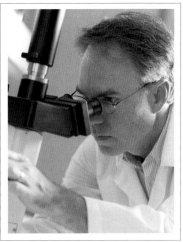

Yosef Yarden, Ph.D., is conducting molecular research at the Weizmann Institute of Science, one of 11 academic centers in Israel supported by PCF funding.

Charles Sawyers, M.D., has used PCF funding at UCLA to discover the pathways of a molecule called "PTEN," known as a tumor suppressor factor.

surrogate markers, Dr. D'Amico was a recipient of the Donald S. Coffey PCF Physician-Scientist Award at the 2003 PCF Scientific Retreat.

Improving quality of life

In the early 1990s, a drug called Atrasentan (formerly designated ABT-627) was being developed by Abbott Laboratories to treat cardiovascular disease. An orally active drug with few side effects, Atrasentan blocks the activity of the molecule endothelin, which closes blood vessels. A team of Johns Hopkins University researchers led by Joel Nelson, M.D., and Michael Carducci, M.D., discovered that endothelin appeared to have a role in prostate cancer growing in bone and in causing pain.

> *"I was a young guy in the field with no track record, but I did have a hypothesis and a little bit of preliminary data to support it,"* Nelson remembers. *"The PCF looked at the idea and said, 'We want to fund this because it's precisely the kind of high-risk, high-gain work that could change the face of things.'"*

Five years of PCF-funded research work paid off by demonstrating that Atrasentan altered the growth of bone metastases. Based on these results, Abbott has committed hundreds of millions of dollars to the ongoing development of Atrasentan to determine whether it can inhibit the growth of prostate cancer cells in bone, relieve pain and improve quality of life for those patients living with the disease. Strategies to gain FDA approval for this indication are being formulated.

"This never would have happened if the PCF had not been willing to think outside the box and give a young investigator the opportunity to spread his wings and test an untested idea," Nelson says. Meanwhile, Nelson's success led him from Johns Hopkins to the University of Pittsburgh, where he became the youngest head of a major urology department in the U.S. when he was appointed in 1999.

Restoring normal patterns

SAHA is a drug discovered at Memorial Sloan-Kettering Cancer Center (MSKCC) and Columbia University that targets histone deacetylases and either stops the growth or causes the death of a broad range of cancer cells. Research on SAHA was conducted by MSKCC President Emeritus Paul Marks, M.D.; Sloan-Kettering Institute Chairman Emeritus Richard Rifkind, M.D.; Victoria Richon, Ph.D., who is currently Director of Biology at Aton Pharma; and Ronald Breslow, Ph.D., a research chemist at Columbia. Preclinical studies directed at prostate cancer were funded in part by the PCF. Results of these studies led to a Phase I clinical trial also partially funded by the PCF and coordinated at MSKCC by Kevin Kelly, D.O., and Howard Scher, M.D.

Imaging

In 1995, John Kurhanewicz, Ph.D., a researcher at the University of California, San Francisco, was developing a new imaging system that would locate metastasized disease and measure its aggressiveness. The PCF's support of his research allowed Kurhanewicz to develop preliminary data that led to more than $3.1 million in NIH grants, and is continuing to lead to new research funding.

"When the Prostate Cancer Foundation funded our initial work it was purely research. We've now been able to take that work into the clinic, and the next step is to make it routine in the clinic," says Kurhanewicz. *"The PCF provided money quickly, with fewer restrictions, so we could go into a whole new area and get data we needed for big government grants.*

"We are now at the point where we can do validation studies in very large populations of men, which will help us understand when to use the exam, when not to, and how individual patients will benefit. Ultimately, we hope to be able to predict how aggressively certain cancers progress and determine how well specific therapies are working."

Short-circuiting cancer growth

Neal Rosen, M.D., Ph.D., a cancer researcher at Sloan-Kettering, was studying the anticancer activity of geldanamycin, an anti-fungal compound. With seed funds from the PCF, Dr. Rosen demonstrated that geldanamycin treatment of cancer cells destroyed molecules that send signals for uncontrolled growth.

A derivative of geldanamycin is being studied in a Sloan-Kettering clinic by Dr. Howard Scher and colleagues. This program is another example of how PCF resources are providing near-term patient benefits by quickly moving promising compounds from the laboratory to a clinical setting.

A lethal payload

One of the earliest PCF-supported research projects helped lead to a greater understanding of PSMA (prostate-specific membrane antigen). Unlike the enzyme PSA, which circulates in the blood, PSMA is a protein expressed on the cell surface of virtually all prostate cancer cells. Neil Bander, M.D., from the New York Hospital, Cornell Medical Center, produced monoclonal anti-bodies to PSMA that bind to living cells and are being used to deliver lethal payloads, such as radioactive molecules and toxins, to prostate cancer cells in patients.

PSMA antibodies are now being developed for the treatment of advanced prostate cancer at three companies: Millennium Pharmaceuticals, Cytogen/Progenics and Medarex. While development is still at an early stage, initial results are encouraging and the Food and Drug Administration granted fast-track review status to the Millennium compound late in 2003. Then, in early 2004, the FDA selected the product as the one oncology drug from among all such drugs in development to pilot a new approvals process that may speed the drug-development timeline. This selection was based on encouraging Phase I data and potential for future benefit to patients.

Apoptosis

Normal, healthy cells maintain a dynamic balance between growth and death. Organs preserve their size and functions because as old cells die, new cells emerge to take their place. In cancer, this balance is disrupted. The cancer cells don't die, and new healthy cells don't thrive.

PCF-sponsored researchers, led by John Reed, M.D., Ph.D., president of the Burnham Institute in San Diego, have studied the ways that cells are programmed to die, a process called apoptosis. Advances from the Burnham Institute study have produced many targets and leads for cancer therapy that, in Dr. Reed's words, "encourage cancer cells to commit suicide" using the body's normal genetic stimulus for cell death. One experimental treatment emerging from this work is in a Phase II clinical trial for prostate cancer. Dr. Reed's discoveries have also suggested diagnostic tests that could predict whether cancer patients will or will not relapse after receiving therapy, providing much-needed information in planning optimal medical management.

Reed's work has become a benchmark in the understanding of apoptosis in all forms of cancer. In fact, for the past decade, he was the world's most-cited scientist in the field of apoptosis according to the Institute for Scientific Information. Dr. Reed was also the world's most-cited scientist in all fields of research for two consecutive years. Reed's success has helped develop a burgeoning scientific community in San Diego.

Fast-tracking the research

Velcade, one of a class of drugs called proteasome inhibitors, has shown strong early indications that it may be effective in treating prostate cancer and other solid tumors. The U.S. Food and Drug Administration has already approved it, following an expedited "priority review," as an injection for the treatment of advanced multiple myeloma. Clinical trials of Velcade, which is marketed by Millennium Pharmaceuticals, are continuing to establish its efficacy in prostate cancer.

Early in its development, Velcade was thought to be a treatment for arthritis and inflammation. Julian Adams, Ph.D., now the chief science officer at Infinity Pharmaceuticals, was convinced that the compound could also treat cancer. But Adams lacked funding to develop this theory. Armed with some "very impressive data," Adams met with Christopher Logothetis, M.D., who heads the prostate cancer research program at the M.D. Anderson Cancer Center in Houston. Logothetis, who has received multiple research awards from the PCF, was quick to see its potential, and arranged a meeting with PCF representatives. The meeting resulted in PCF funding of a small clinical trial of Velcade in cancer and generated investor interest in the program.

> *"Our mechanism was very novel and counter-intuitive. But the PCF had the vision to fund us through M.D. Anderson so that we could build a compelling case,"* Adams says. *"And once we were ready for clinical trials, the PCF again stepped in with increasingly larger grants. But even more importantly, they helped convince the National Cancer Institute to let us fast-track our research."*

The development of Velcade has all the hallmarks of the PCF's approach: initial funding of an innovative idea; leveraging its investment by attracting larger federal grants; and working with bio-pharmaceutical companies to accelerate approval of the drug and get it to market.

Tumor suppression

Charles Sawyers, M.D., at the University of California, Los Angeles, has studied the molecule "PTEN," known as a tumor suppressor factor. Mutations in PTEN are associated with aggressive prostate cancer, and Sawyers has used his PCF funding to discover the pathways regulated by the molecule. An October 2003 *Wall Street Journal* article quoted Sawyers as saying, "I'm enthusiastic about targeting this gene pathway … big pharma, small pharma, biotech and the cancer world are all over [it]." There is optimism that this work could lead to novel therapeutic interventions for advanced prostate cancer.

Filling the pipeline

Over the past decade, early development of several other promising drug candidates was funded in part by the PCF:

- AstraZeneca has advanced Iressa (EGF receptor tyrosine kinase inhibitor) into clinical development for advanced prostate cancer. This drug has already been approved for the treatment of selected patients with advanced non-small-cell lung cancer.

- Novartis has obtained approval for Zometa, a third generation bisphosphonate for the preservation of bone mineral density in men undergoing long-term hormone treatment for prostate cancer.

- With leadership from Johns Hopkins University, Cell Genesys is developing a gene therapy viral vector that selectively replicates in and kills prostate cancer cells.

- Work by leaders in the PCF Therapy Consortium contributed to the development of taxane-based chemotherapy regimens. Aventis Pharmaceuticals is now in late-stage clinical development of Taxotere, a taxane, for advanced prostate cancer. Members of the Consortium are optimistic that with FDA review, this regimen will be approved.

This progress has occurred in areas where there was little innovative clinical research a decade ago. Biotech and pharmaceutical company executives agree that the PCF has been primarily responsible for opening the research floodgates.

"Everybody talks about facilitating engagement and collaboration across academia, industry, and government agencies," says Perry Nisen, M.D., Ph.D., divisional vice president of global oncology development at Abbott Laboratories. *"But who actually accomplishes it in a demonstrable and meaningful way? The Prostate Cancer Foundation does. The PCF spans the whole gamut of clinical care, nutrition, policy, connections into legislation, economics and healthcare. It's unique."*

Owen Witte, M.D., a renowned UCLA researcher who received an award from the Milken Family Foundation earlier in his career (see Chapter 1) and has since received multiple research awards from the PCF and others, concurs with Dr. Nisen's assessment:

"The quality of science proposed has gone up logarithmically over the past decade and I think that's a very good sign because what it means is that better and better people are asking better and better questions. It's taken their game up, and the PCF's game has taken the whole field up in addition to its own quality."

In 2003, a team at Johns Hopkins University that includes urological surgeon Patrick Walsh, M.D., oncologist William Nelson, M.D., Ph.D., pathologist Angelo DeMarzo, M.D. and urological geneticist William Isaacs, Ph.D., published an important review article on prostate cancer in the *New England Journal of Medicine*. Walsh, one of the most famous urologists in America, wrote to Milken:

"This pioneering manuscript would not have been possible without the magnificent support you've provided for our multidisciplinary team of scientists. You recognized that to solve this problem at its root cause required the talents of scientists with diverse backgrounds. We would not have been able to attract and retain the critical mass of investigators who put this concept together without your support … You have been our partner in this process of discovery and I hope you share in our pleasure at the progress of our work."

Assessing the Impact

In the decade since the Prostate Cancer Foundation was established, the number of American men who die each year from prostate cancer has fallen, the number of men who receive PSA tests has risen, and the organization has become the world's largest philanthropic source of funds for prostate cancer research.

Perhaps the best way to assess the PCF's impact is simply to let leading doctors and scientists who have been involved in PCF programs put it in their own words. Here's some of what they said, recorded in a series of interviews during 2003:

> *"The Prostate Cancer Foundation has done more than any other organization to reduce deaths from prostate cancer. By funding the best and brightest scientists, the PCF has helped launch new approaches to advanced disease and attracted young vigorous investigators to spend their life pursuing them. History will show that the field of investigation in prostate cancer bloomed when the PCF began."*
>
> Patrick C. Walsh, M.D.
> Johns Hopkins University

> *"We set out to achieve some incredibly ambitious goals with the Prostate Cancer Foundation. We wanted to do no less than change the paradigm of medical research; to raise the public's awareness; to get academics, industry and government collaborating more effectively; to increase federal*

research funding; and more. When you consider that the PCF has put close to $150 million into research and you think about the drugs that have emerged from that research, it would be the most successful biotechnology firm in the world if it were a private company. I never could have imagined the success we've had."

Stuart Holden, M.D.
Cedars-Sinai Medical Center
Medical Director, Prostate Cancer Foundation

"The effect the PCF has had on the entire field of prostate cancer research is really immeasurable. They've transformed prostate cancer research from a neglected small field to a major interest of the scientific community, the pharmaceutical industry and Congress."

Pinchas Cohen, M.D.
University of California, Los Angeles

"As somebody who was involved in the PCF fairly early on, what I see today is amazing. I'm not aware of any private organization that has had such a tremendous impact on a particular discipline or field of study as the PCF has in such a short period of time.

"Attending the (PCF) Scientific Retreat is a little like drinking from a fire hose. The problem isn't that there isn't enough information, but it clearly tests the capacity of any one person to drink it all in. It's the place where you learn about what's coming down the pike. It's like putting your ear to the rail before you actually hear the train coming – it's where you first hear rumblings about what will be in the public domain two or three years later."

Joel Nelson, M.D.
University of Pittsburgh

"History will show that Michael Milken launched the campaign to defeat prostate cancer through supporting basic and clinical research and creating essential infrastructure and resources. He has done more than any other single individual to advance this cause. His impact will be felt for years to come as the projects supported through his efforts bear fruit."

William J. Catalona, M.D.
Northwestern University

"No one has articulated the greatness of the human spirit like Mike Milken does. Somehow in his presence, it looks like everything is possible."

Moshe Shike, M.D.
Memorial Sloan-Kettering Cancer Center

"The Prostate Cancer Foundation has changed the face of prostate cancer research. Chemotherapy was once viewed as ineffective and an unpopular therapy option. Because of the PCF's approach and willingness to fund our studies, we have been able to demonstrate its effectiveness."

Christopher J. Logothetis, M.D.
M.D. Anderson Cancer Center

"The Prostate Cancer Foundation has helped further the search for a cure for prostate cancer through its financial support and by fostering a sense of community among scientists, doctors, patients and families. The PCF's unique funding mechanism has helped researchers pursue their work with greater autonomy, lessening their financial burdens and paperwork, which would otherwise interfere with their time, concentration and energy. I've been able to pursue independent novel research projects, and establish a diverse network of people. And the PCF always reminds me of the very

human aspect of the kinds of that science we conduct in the laboratory."

June Chan, Sc.D.
Harvard School of Public Health

"A decade ago, prostate cancer was rarely discussed. Men were just learning about a new blood test (for PSA) and becoming curious and concerned about the disease. For many men with advanced prostate cancer, curiosity and concern about the disease were replaced by dread and despair. Over the past several years, through the efforts of Michael Milken and the Prostate Cancer Foundation, new hope has arisen. Chemotherapy has been refined. New drugs are on the horizon. Immunotherapy has gained a foothold. Gene therapies are in clinical trials. Anti-progression and anti-angiogenesis drugs are on the horizon. The role of diet as a therapeutic adjunct is under scrutiny. I have always believed that prostate cancer, and all other cancers, can be cured. Michael Milken shares that belief. As an advocate, his belief in a cure for prostate cancer is accompanied by an impatience that has become his inspiration. Mike has provided inspiration for all who labor to cure prostate cancer."

William G. Nelson, M.D., Ph.D.
Johns Hopkins University

"We have to take risky steps in terms of drug development and patient care, and the Prostate Cancer Foundation gives us the freedom to go outside the box. Even more important, the PCF has brought together the resources of other researchers, investigators and clinicians in a support system to take these risky steps. If I'm in the middle of a trial, I know I can count on M.D. Anderson, Sloan-Kettering and others to say, 'Yeah, this is the right way to do it.' That network has really allowed this field to develop.

"The PCF has validated the prostate cancer field. Biotech and pharmaceutical companies have realized there's a market here, and researchers now know that it makes sense to have a career in our field. When I got into prostate cancer, it was a risk. Now there's no risk. It's great. Ten years ago, prostate cancer was a bad word to biotech and pharmaceutical companies. Nobody had really validated prostate cancer as a model to develop drugs. All the drugs under development were going to those areas where the model had been validated – breast cancer, lung cancer and others. The PCF came along and set the framework for prostate cancer."

David B. Agus, M.D.
Cedars-Sinai Medical Center

"When I was a young clinician/investigator, the PCF provided me with probably the most important opportunity of my career by allowing me to think freely."

Guillermo Garcia-Manero, M.D.
University of Texas

"The Prostate Cancer Foundation has increased awareness among the public through fundraising events and media efforts. Nearly every patient entering the clinic is now aware of the PCF, and many have information on prostate cancer provided by the Foundation. They've also influenced the thinking of decision makers in Washington to ensure their recognition of the seriousness of this disease as a major public health problem that needs more research funding. And through its own funding mechanism, it has stimulated hundreds of research ideas that investigators can present for funding in streamlined format, as well as receive support in a matter of weeks after submission of their application. This process is the most efficient and rapid mechanism to obtain support for prostate cancer research."

George Wilding, M.D.
University of Wisconsin

"No one has done more to increase the quality and the impact of prostate cancer research than Mike Milken. No one. Mike deserves huge credit for what he has accomplished and it's quite remarkable. I can take any other disease issue that you might want to think about – AIDS, breast cancer, and so on – and there are many, many people putting effort into it. But if you ask in the prostate cancer world, 'Who outside of the biomedical establishment has had an impact?' I think immediately you would come up with Mike Milken."

Owen Witte, M.D.
UCLA

"Mike Milken demonstrated that we didn't have to accept the status quo, that we could jump start better research and more research into cancer and use prostate as an example. And that we could develop consensus among people, both in and out of government, that could make a tremendous difference in terms of increasing the chances that someday we will reach a major historical event."

Paul H. Lange, M.D.
University of Washington

"There is a tremendous delay from the time things happen in the lab until they are recognized by a wider circle of scientists, and other people begin to say, 'Hey, this might be worth looking at.' The PCF has brought the best basic science minds into the field and they're beginning to understand it, making important contributions, with new ideas percolating up that we can then take to the bedside and begin to try and find new and better ways to treat patients. This is what being a doctor is all about – finding new hope to give to patients."

Peter Scardino, M.D.
Memorial Sloan-Kettering Cancer Center

"As a former member of the PCF board, I can tell you that the organization has one overriding uniqueness: Mike Milken. Mike created awareness where there was none; he single-handedly stimulated a cascade of NCI funding; he got doctors and scientists to go into the field; and he raised awareness of the crucial importance of clinical trials – many more patients now enter trials. As a result, patients have a choice of many more therapies and more effective therapies today."

John H. Glick, M.D.
University of Pennsylvania Cancer Center

"Mike Milken with his vision of the future recognized that cancer was not just a scientific problem or a medical problem, but that it was an economic problem, a political problem, a cultural problem and a social problem. And that kind of vision, that kind of leadership, I personally think is why God has gifted him with the ability to be with us over these past ten years to provide the kind of leadership to bring us together for a societal solution to the problem of cancer."

Andrew von Eschenbach, M.D.
National Cancer Institute

Looking to the Future

On January 20, 2004, Mike Milken stood before one of the most distinguished gatherings of cancer experts in the world. He was about to deliver the keynote address to a Leadership Round-table convened by the National Cancer Institute in Washington. It was a select audience of only about 80 people, but it included senior representatives from several of the largest companies in the world – General Electric, IBM, Intel, Pfizer, Johnson & Johnson – plus several other major pharmaceutical and biotechnology firms – Eli Lilly, Novartis, Amgen and more; the NCI's Director and senior management, officials from the White House Office of Science and Technology Policy, the Department of Homeland Security and the Food and Drug Administration; a Nobel laureate; and the heads of virtually every Comprehensive Cancer Center in the U.S.

There were several old friends in the audience: Lee Hood (see Chapter 6); Jonathan Simons (Chapters 3 and 4); Anna Barker, who had organized the Roundtable for the NCI (Chapter 7); Steve Case, founder of America Online and co-founder of Accelerate Brain Cancer Cure; and Stephen Fodor, chairman and co-founder of Affymetrix – a leader in applying the principles of semicon-ductor technology to the life sciences – whom Mike had met a decade earlier while touring major companies working on advanced therapeutics.

The two-day Roundtable was convened with the goal of devel-oping new strategies for reducing the nation's cancer burden, especially though public/private/academic collaborations that could focus strategic technology resources most effectively. It produced, in the words of the NCI Director, "a wealth of substantive solutions" that should help accelerate the war on cancer. But standing at the podium that cold January day, Milken saw in the assembled faces the history of the Prostate Cancer Foundation. These leaders from various fields were at the forefront of technologies and research approaches that the PCF had been encouraging since 1993. And they were harnessing new approaches like nanotechnology and artificial intelligence that had not previously been employed in the War on Cancer. It was a stunning affirmation of a mission and strategy that began with some notes scribbled on an airplane more than a decade earlier.

A few weeks later, Milken and PCF CEO Leslie Michelson spoke to a Prostate Cancer Roundtable organized by the Majority Leader of the New York State Senate in Albany. The purpose of this gathering was to develop support for a bill that would allow New York taxpayers to check a box on their state tax returns directing that their refunds be sent to a non-profit organization funding prostate cancer research. The Majority Leader, Senator Joseph Bruno, who is a prostate cancer survivor, introduced Milken:

> *"The more you learn about Mike Milken, the more impressed you get. I am amazed what he has done. Of course, the Milken Family Foundation has directed hundreds of millions of dollars into research on cancer and other serious diseases. But in my mind, Mike's greatest value is as a role model for people doing something on a continuous basis to help people. A lot of wealthy people take pleasure in writing checks. Mike is different. He spends his personal time and energy. Thanks to his commitment, we are going to do some great things to improve the quality of life for people here in New York State, and consequently throughout the United States and the world."*

Later that day, the New York State Senate passed the tax check-off bill by the unprecedented vote of 60-0.

Once again, it was clear that the PCF concept, conceived 11 years earlier, was having a major impact. It had set out to increase resources for all medical research, to bring greater focus to cancer research, and to accelerate progress against prostate cancer in particular. It has achieved all three of these goals. In the process, it has created a new model for funding medical research (Chapter 3) that has been adopted by other organizations; it has raised awareness of the need for greater government funding (Chapter 5) and of the need for individuals to get tested (Chapters 6, 9 and 10); it has strengthened collaboration among major medical institutions (Chapter 8); it has focused medical professionals and patients on the importance of prevention, especially through nutrition, that could reduce the expected growth rate of disease (Chapter 11); and, most important, it has funded the development of important new therapies (Chapter 12).

There are far more drug candidates in the pipeline for use in prostate cancer than ever before – 50 percent more than just five years ago. Many of these drugs will eventually be approved and will have an enormously positive effect on patients. The challenge is not a lack of opportunities; it is continuing to develop the resources and public will to accelerate development of all the opportunities and offer more hope to the two million American men currently suffering with prostate cancer and the three million more who could be diagnosed in the next decade as the baby boomers age.

In fact, despite all the progress to date, current projections suggest that the incidence of prostate cancer will increase sharply in coming decades unless there are major new break-throughs.

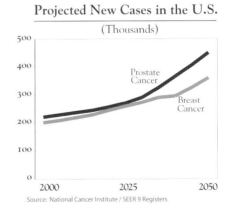

Projected New Cases in the U.S.

(Thousands)

Prostate Cancer

Breast Cancer

2000   2025   2050

Source: National Cancer Institute / SEER 9 Registers

As increasing numbers of men reach the target age for prostate cancer, beginning at age 50, the number diagnosed will increase to 300,000 and annual deaths could reach 50,000 by 2015. That means that this disease is the cancer with the largest expected increase in the next decade.

Accelerating medical solutions

Clearly, much remains to be done. But PCF-supported researchers are optimistic. Consider the enthusiasm of David Agus, M.D., research director of the Louis Warschaw Prostate Cancer Center at Cedars-Sinai Medical Center in Los Angeles:

> "The outlook is great. We have exciting new technologies that will help us personalize treatments for each individual. For the first time, I can see hope through the patient's eyes. I've got effective new drugs, and I've got hope that I'll have better drugs in six months, and better drugs six months after that. I can see a pipeline where I can hopefully make this a chronic disease."

Milken addressed this acceleration of technology in a July 2003 article on the editorial page of *The Wall Street Journal*:

> "Technology that didn't exist five years ago allows us to look at thousands of genes simultaneously. By understanding the differences among these genes, doctors may be able to treat patients effectively years before symptoms appear. According to Dr. Alan Robinson, vice provost for medical education at UCLA, 'There's a major revolution coming in predictive medicine that's as important as the discovery of the germ theory.' The cost of sequencing a single gene has dropped from millions of dollars a quarter-century ago to $150 in 1998 and less than $9 today. Dr. Leroy Hood, president of the Institute for Systems Biology, believes that in 10 years we may be able to sequence an individual's entire genome - more than 20,000 genes - in 20 minutes for less than $1,000."

In the same article, Milken announced the formation of a new organization, FasterCures / The Center for Accelerating Medical Solutions. Unlike the Prostate Cancer Foundation, which funds medical research, FasterCures is a think tank – or, as its staff likes to call it, an *action* tank – dedicated to shortening the time it takes to find cures and better treatments for all serious diseases. Faster-Cures is mobilizing economists, medical researchers, clinicians, biologists, ethicists, genomics specialists, chemists, physicists, mathematicians, computer scientists, legislative analysts and others to evaluate the entire research and treatment process, publish concrete policy recommendations, and provide leadership for their implementation. The goal is to find new efficiencies that can accelerate scientific discovery while reducing misplaced priorities, sometimes inefficient regulations, and conflicting incentives that slow progress.

Greg Simon, the President of FasterCures, draws an analogy to rail transportation. *"We have the technology to build 300-mile-per-hour trains that could speed from Washington to New York in an hour. The problem is that the tracks are inadequate, forcing even the fastest trains to slow down below 100 miles per hour. In medical research, we have superb technology and the world's best scientists. But we throw roadblocks in their path, which delays development of cures. FasterCures is committed to 'laying new track' in the health sciences sector."*

If progress in medical research someday eliminates the burden of cancer, all of humanity will benefit from the reduction in suffering. And the economic benefits would be immense. University of Chicago economists Kevin Murphy and Robert Topel estimate an $800 billion a year savings in the U.S. alone and much more worldwide. That kind of potential return, multiplied by the potential inherent in defeating other serious diseases, is the *raison d'être* of FasterCures.

Milken's *Wall Street Journal* article explained the importance of the FasterCures mission:

> "More than a million Americans suffer heart attacks every year. Strokes hit 600,000. Cancer kills 550,000. Our children face a greater risk of dying from cancer than their grandparents faced. Even a single year's acceleration in medical solutions would make a big difference. For example, finding a breast-cancer cure just one year earlier could prevent hundreds of thousands of deaths worldwide among women whose disease is still at a curable stage, and save millions more from painful, disfiguring treatments.
>
> "The choice is ours. We can sit back and wait for more cures and better treatments, or we can marshal our resources to solve medical problems sooner and save more lives. Maybe yours."

Epilogue

Early in 2004, Mike Milken reflected on what the Prostate Cancer Foundation has meant:

> "It's eleven years since I was diagnosed and I hardly know where to begin in expressing my thanks, not only for my own good health, but also for the skill and perseverance of all the PCF-supported medical researchers whose work offers hope to millions of others. Thousands of people around the world have done so much to achieve the PCF's goals. The members of the board of directors have been magnificent in guiding our mission; the PCF staff has been indefatigable. Hundreds of athletes, artists, entertainers and public officials have pitched in to help. These examples inspire all of us to rededicate ourselves to the quest for a world without cancer.

> "On a personal note, it has undoubtedly been therapeutic for me to immerse myself in all the PCF's many initiatives over the past decade. Everyone I've asked to help – whether with money, time, talent or other resources – has cooperated wonderfully. That has been the best medicine of all."

Some Highlights of the Prostate Cancer Foundation's First Decade

1993

- After two decades of supporting medical research, Mike Milken is diagnosed with advanced prostate cancer and establishes the Prostate Cancer Foundation (originally called CaP CURE) as a public charity.

- Stuart (Skip) Holden, M.D., becomes the PCF's medical director; Allen Flans becomes executive director.

- The Milken Family Foundation commits $25 million over five years (later renewed with a second $25 million commitment), a professional staff is hired and a 15-member Board of Directors convenes.

- The PCF establishes its groundbreaking awards process, which limits applications to five pages and funds approved research applications within 90 days.

- The first 30 competitive research award winners receive $4.5 million in grants.

- The PCF makes the first of five grants to Judah Folkman, M.D. (Harvard Medical School) to continue his work in the area of anti-angiogenesis. Folkman's work will influence not only prostate cancer research, but nearly every branch of oncology.

- The PCF hosts its first Call-to-Action Dinner at the U.S. Capitol to honor 1993 award winners.

- Industrialist John Kluge hosts a seminal roundtable meeting about prostate cancer research and funding at his Charlottesville, Virginia, farm.

1994

- Former Presidents Ford, Carter, Reagan and Bush join the PCF's Presidential Honorary Board.

- The PCF's first New York fund-raising dinner, hosted by Bill Cosby, is held at the 21 Club. President Clinton calls to congratulate the PCF on its contributions to medical research.

- Supporters as diverse as Los Angeles Mayor Richard Riordan and Terry Semel, now chairman of Yahoo!, learn more about prostate cancer at a PCF educational/fund-raising event at Pickfair in Los Angeles.

- Milken emphasizes the opportunities in prostate cancer research at the National Biotechnology Conference.

- Neil Bander, M.D., produces monoclonal antibodies to PSMA (Prostate Specific Membrane Antigen) that bind to living cells. As of 2003, three companies are testing these antibodies to develop treatments for advanced prostate cancer patients.

- Nearly 100 scientists and physicians attend the PCF's first annual Scientific Retreat in Santa Barbara.

- The PCF's scientific review panel awards $4.8 million to 46 competitive award winners.

- Several Congressional leaders attend the second Capitol Hill Call-to-Action Dinner.

1995

- PCF-funded researchers hold a Tissue Bank Summit to establish protocols for harvesting prostate-cancer tissue.

- Richard (Rick) Atkins, M.D., is named executive director of the PCF.

- The PCF makes initial investments in four regional tissue banks and the Gene and Family Studies Consortium.

- The PCF coordinates a Working Meeting on Standards in Washington to accelerate the release of oncology drugs.

- Joel Nelson, M.D., and Michael Carducci, M.D., use PCF funding to discover that a cardiovascular disease drug, Atrasentan, may be helpful for prostate cancer patients. (See 2000.)
- More than 130 physicians and scientists attend the PCF's second annual Scientific Retreat, which features more than 60 presentations.
- The PCF funds Dr. Jonathan Simons at Johns Hopkins University, who will develop GVAX, a promising anti-prostate cancer vaccine.
- Elaine and Steve Wynn host the first Shadow Creek Invitational Golf Tournament to benefit the PCF.
- Milken, General Norman Schwarzkopf, Stuart Holden, M.D, and Leroy Hood, M.D., Ph.D., appear on CNN's *Larry King Live* to discuss a prostate-cancer family study, and more than 3,000 callers from 18 countries phone in to learn more.
- The PCF organizes the National Cancer Summit in Washington; Milken presents a 10-point plan to rethink the war on cancer. (See Appendix C.)
- The PCF presents $10.2 million to 62 competitive award winners at its third Call-to-Action Dinner in Washington.
- General Schwarzkopf is honored at the PCF's New York dinner.
- PCF-funded researcher John Kurhanewicz, Ph.D. (University of California, San Francisco), develops a new imaging system that locates metastasized disease and measures its aggressiveness.
- Lynda and Stewart Resnick host a highly successful West Coast fund-raising dinner.

1996

- With PCF input, President Clinton signs an executive order to fast-track cancer drugs.
- The PCF Therapy Consortium is launched to coordinate research at leading U.S. cancer centers.

- Following more than 100 Congressional visits by PCF board members, led by Intel Chairman Andy Grove, Congress approves a Prostate Cancer Research Program in the Department of Defense with an initial appropriation of $45 million.

- *Time* magazine puts General Schwarzkopf on its cover for an article about prostate cancer.

- Intel and Hewlett-Packard hardware and software donations help distant PCF researchers collaborate.

- PCF-funded Dr. Charles Sawyers (UCLA) discovers new pathways of cancer development in a tumor suppressor factor molecule.

- *Fortune* magazine cover features PCF board member Andy Grove, who details the story of his prostate cancer diagnosis and treatment.

- Milken, Dr. David Heber and Olivia Newton-John discuss nutrition on *Larry King Live*.

- The PCF hosts its first Nutritional Summit.

- The PCF sponsors awareness days and activities with Major League Baseball teams, the predecessor of the Home Run Challenge.

- PCF researcher John Reed, M.D., Ph.D. (Burnham Institute, San Diego), develops benchmark understanding of apoptosis (cell death), which has led to potential new treatments for all forms of cancer.

- The PCF helps form and fund the National Prostate Cancer Coalition (NPCC).

- Milken is joined by California Senator Barbara Boxer in speaking to more than 1,300 prostate cancer survivors at a Southern California conference in Buena Park.

- The PCF helps establish the UCLA Center for Human Nutrition under David Heber, M.D., Ph.D.

- PCF-funded studies by Paul Marks, M.D., Victoria Richon, Ph.D., and others show that SAHA stops the growth of or kills cancer cells. The PCF later funds clinical trials of SAHA at Memorial Sloan-Kettering Cancer Center by Howard Scher, M.D.

- The PCF Scientific Retreat is held at Lake Tahoe for the first time.

- The PCF brings together the parties needed to establish a center of excellence in prostate cancer at the University of California, San Francisco.

- The PCF awards a total of $13.8 million grants in 1996, including $750,000 to the Nutrition Project.

- At the request of Florida Senator Connie Mack, Milken addresses nearly 500 prostate cancer survivors in Orlando.

1997

- Former U.S. Senator and presidential candidate Bob Dole makes a TV public service announcement for the PCF.

- Milken and testicular cancer survivor Lance Armstrong speak at the 5th Annual Genitourinary Oncology Conference at the M.D. Anderson Cancer Center.

- The PCF publishes the *Nutrition & Prostate Cancer* monograph.

- The first PCF/Major League Baseball Home Run Challenge (HRC) to raise funds for research garners widespread print and broadcast coverage in cities around the country.

- Milken urges more cancer research funding at a Montgomery Securities investment conference.

- The PCF annual Scientific Retreat has 200 attendees and 87 presentations. The *Journal of the American Medical Association* calls it a "major event" of the war on cancer.

- Milken makes the first of several appearances on *The Charlie Rose Show*.

- A *Los Angeles Times* article says, *"It used to be an issue men refused to talk about. Now prostate cancer is a hot topic."*

- PCF Board Member Sue Gin tells a White House roundtable discussion that prostate cancer research needs more funding.

- Milken provides prostate cancer research updates at the American Society for Therapeutic Radiology and Oncology conference in Los Angeles, and at the Scripps/San Diego Business Journal Healthcare 2000 conference.

- The PCF is added to the Health & Fitness section of America Online (AOL).

- Milken, Ellen Stovall, others appear on *Larry King Live* to announce THE MARCH.

- The PCF's scientific review panel announces $16 million will fund 85 research awards.

1998

- Lynne and Mickey Tarnopol host the PCF New York Dinner, filling the ballroom at the Waldorf Astoria with nearly 1,100 contributors.

- Donald Trump hosts the first Pro/Am Tennis Invitational at the Mar-a-Lago Club in Palm Beach to benefit the PCF's prostate cancer research programs. It's later renamed the Carl H. Lindner Tennis Invitational.

- The PCF establishes Young Investigator Awards, providing six, three-year $150,000 research grants.

- Reggie Jackson and Milken promote the PCF/Major League Baseball Home Run Challenge on national TV.

- THE MARCH, with heavy PCF involvement, draws 500,000 marchers to 200 cities and the National Mall.

- The PCF Scientific Retreat at Lake Tahoe is biggest ever event and features presentation of clinical results from a PSMA monoclonal antibody therapy.

- With seed funds from the PCF, Neal Rosen, M.D., Ph.D., demonstrates that geldanamycin destroys molecules that cause prostate cancer growth.

- *The Taste for Living Cookbook: Mike Milken's Favorite Recipes for Fighting Cancer* is published.

- With PCF input, Congress requires the National Institutes of Health to develop a five-year prostate cancer research investment strategy.

- *Newsweek* mentions the PCF in a cover story on "Cancer & Diet: Eating to Beat the Odds."

- R.D. and Joan Dale Hubbard, with Senior Tour golfer Jim Colbert, inaugurate the Benefit at BIGHORN golf tournament.
- The PCF awards nearly $18 million to fund 81 competitive research awards.

1999

- Senior PGA TOUR for the CURE begins, and is featured at 43 events during the year.
- In a cover story, *BusinessWeek* says Milken "has done more to advance the cause" of cancer research than anyone.
- As urged by the PCF, the U.S. Postal Service issues a prostate cancer awareness stamp.
- Milken joins Yankees manager Joe Torre and former Senator Bob Dole to testify before a U.S. Senate Subcommittee on cancer funding; then they appear on *Larry King Live*.
- PCF-funded researchers at Johns Hopkins announce a vaccine to strengthen the immune system against prostate cancer.
- Molecular and cell biologist James Allison, Ph.D., (University of California, Berkeley) uses PCF funding to study the CTLA-4 molecule. Monoclonal antibodies to CTLA-4 help new cancer vaccines work more effectively.
- Steve and Elaine Wynn and Joe Torre are honored at the PCF's New York Dinner, as Sting and Paul Simon entertain.

2000

- President Clinton names PCF Board Member Michael Phelps winner of the Enrico Fermi Award.
- Abbott Labs takes Atrasentan into Phase III trials to determine if it inhibits prostate cancer in bones, relieves pain and improves quality of life for prostate cancer patients. Atrasentan was first studied in prostate cancer with PCF funding.
- *U.S. News & World Report*: "[The PCF's] work is making a difference and has led to 70 human clinical trials."
- President Clinton requires the Health Care Financing

Administration to cover routine patient costs in clinical trials as previously urged by the PCF.

- The PCF joins the U.S. Conference of Mayors to promote greater awareness of prostate cancer.

- Milken stresses the importance of the biotechnology industry in a keynote speech to 5,000 attendees at the eHealthcare World conference.

- The PCF provides information at both major political parties' conventions. The GOP urges more PSA testing. Vice President Gore calls for doubling the nation's commitment to biomedical research.

- Milken gives major speeches at the University of Sydney and at the Peter MacCallum Cancer Centre in Australia urging internationalization of cancer research.

- Attendance at the 7th annual Scientific Retreat in Lake Tahoe grows to more than 300.

2001

- The PCF's Howard Soule, Ph.D. joins the Department of Defense's Prostate Cancer Research Program Integration Panel, succeeding Stuart Holden, M.D.

- The FDA approves Novartis' new drug, Zometa, for treating prostate cancer and other solid tumors. Early research funded by the PCF is a crucial contribution.

- The 2001 PCF/Major League Baseball Home Run Challenge raises $2.25 million for prostate cancer research.

- Safeway Corp. launches a new customer and employee donation campaign to benefit prostate cancer, raising $750,000, a total that will grow to nearly $5 million by 2004.

- Milken appears on the *Rush Limbaugh Show* to discuss prostate cancer in America. Thousands of listeners sign on to www.mikemilken.com for more information.

- California Governor Davis signs legislation promoted by the PCF requiring health insurance companies and Medi-Cal to pay for clinical trials' costs.

- The PCF hosts the first Gourmet Games fund-raising event

at Bill Tilley's Hollywood home, drawing more than 100 business leaders, researchers and celebrities to compete in wine- and food-tasting competitions.

- The PCF New York Dinner honors the Mack brothers and New York Fire Department firefighters, and eulogizes recently deceased board member Leslie Misrock.

2002

- Milken discusses the effect obesity and lifestyle decisions can play in prostate cancer and other serious diseases at the Art and Science of Health Promotion annual conference.

- Phyllis and Dennis Washington host the first Indian Wells Invitational Tennis Tournament, with proceeds to support PCF research.

- Leslie Michelson becomes PCF Vice Chairman and CEO.

- The Milken Institute annual Global Conference expands the number of panels addressing medical issues and features several PCF-funded researchers.

- The PCF Home Run Challenge is named one of the few official partners of Major League Baseball.

- The PCF's Scientific Retreat returns to Washington, D.C., where members of Congress and the head of the National Cancer Institute address 325 prominent scientists.

- In Israel, the PCF funds a center of excellence award that coordinates research at leading institutes.

- Milken visits Munekado Kojima, M.D., director of the Nagoya Urology Hospital in Japan, to discuss the effects of different diets on prostate cancer in Japan and the U.S.

- The 2nd annual Los Angeles Gourmet Games moves to Santa Monica and attracts 120 business leaders, researchers and celebrities.

- Harvard researcher Anthony D'Amico publishes a study with PCF support showing that a doubling of a man's PSA score in three months is a strong statistical predictor of death from prostate cancer.

- The PCF participates in the National Dialogue on Cancer (now C-Change) in Washington, D.C.

2003

- Millennium Pharmaceuticals gets FDA approval for Velcade, a proteasome inhibitor that was studied with PCF funding in Phase I with the help of PCF-funded researcher Christopher Logothetis, M.D. (M.D. Anderson Cancer Center).

- Work by leaders in the PCF Therapy Consortium contributes to the development of taxane-based chemotherapy regimens for advanced prostate cancer. Aventis Pharmaceuticals develops Taxotere for use in prostate cancer.

- The Prostate Cancer Foundation unveils its new name and logo, replacing CaP CURE.

- With early PCF funding and researcher involvement in clinical trials, AstraZeneca takes Iressa, an EGF receptor tyrosine kinase inhibitor, into clinical development for advanced prostate cancer.

- Milken discusses the need for accelerating the pace of medical science at the annual Pharmaceutical Research and Manufacturers of America (PhRMA) conference.

- At the Milken Institute Global Conference, Milken announces FasterCures / The Center for Accelerating Medical Solutions, dedicated to finding faster cures for all serious diseases.

- Drs. Jonathan Simons, Leland Chung and others share a $10-million Department of Defense grant for work growing out of previous PCF-funded research.

- Joining prostate cancer research advocate Harry Belafonte and Charles "Snuffy" Myers, M.D., at the Prostate Cancer Research Institute's annual conference, Milken emphasizes lifestyle actions that survivors can take to improve and extend their quality of life.

- George Clooney, Matt Damon and Sugar Ray Leonard support the PCF by attending the eighth annual Shadow Creek golf tournament.

- H.J. Heinz Corp. joins the growing list of sponsors for the PCF Home Run Challenge (HRC); funds raised for the HRC since its inception exceed $18 million.

- Milken and Peter Carroll, M.D., chairman of the UCSF Department of Urology, speak about an expected increase in prostate cancer diagnoses at the Aspen Center for Integrative Health.

- PCF-funded researchers at Johns Hopkins publish an important review article on prostate cancer in the *New England Journal of Medicine*.

- PCF funding of research programs at 11 academic centers in Israel reaches $4.7 million.

- Cell phone pioneer Craig McCaw and Microsoft's Jim Allchin help inaugurate the Seattle Gourmet Games, followed by the 3rd annual Los Angeles Gourmet Games.

- The 10th annual PCF Scientific Retreat in New York is attended by 350 of the world's leading scientists and physicians, government leaders and patient advocates.

- The New York Dinner marks the 10th anniversary of the Prostate Cancer Foundation and honors Mike and Lori Milken. Cher, Whoopi Goldberg, David Foster, Lionel Richie and Michael Buble entertain.

- Total funding for the Department of Defense Prostate Cancer Research Program (PCRP) since 1996 totals $395 million and has supported 800 peer-reviewed programs. The PCRP now holds its annual meeting at the Milken Institute building in Santa Monica.

- Since 1993, total government funding of prostate cancer research has grown by a factor of 20 to $500 million

- Contributions to the PCF pass the $200 million mark.

- PCF programs from 1993 through 2003 have funded more than 1,100 projects worldwide.

- Annual prostate cancer deaths fall to an estimated 28,900, significantly below expert predictions of a decade earlier.

2004

- The FDA approves Avastin, an anti-angiogenesis drug, for use in treating advanced colon cancer. Further trials of Avastin as a treatment for recurrent prostate cancer are expected.

- Following presentations by the PCF, the New York State Senate unanimously passes a bill that would allow New York taxpayers to check a box on their state tax returns directing that their refunds be sent to a non-profit organization funding prostate cancer research.

- The PCF chairman and president participate in a crucial NCI Leadership Roundtable, which brings executives from several of the largest companies in the world together with top government officials and the heads of major cancer centers to refine America's national strategy for reducing the burden of cancer.

Major Competitive Research Awards by the Prostate Cancer Foundation
1993-2003

(Note: Affiliations are shown at the time of the award and in some cases are not the award recipient's current affiliation.)

Albert Einstein College of Medicine
$75,000
Nicole B. Schreiber-Agus, Ph.D.

Assaf Harofe Medical Center (Israel)
$150,000
Amnon Zisman, M.D.

Bar-Ilan University (Israel)
$225,000
Shlomo Grossman, Ph.D.
Uri Nir, Ph.D.

Baylor University/College of Medicine
$3,200,000
Jacques Banchereau, Ph.D.
Norman M. Greenberg, Ph.D.
Dov Kadmon, M.D.
Paula Kaplan-Lefko, Ph.D.
Michael Kattan, Ph.D.
Dolores J. Lamb, Ph.D.
Bert W. O'Malley, M.D.
David R. Rowley, Ph.D.
Peter T. Scardino, M.D.
Timothy C. Thompson, Ph.D.
Ming-Jer Tsai, Ph.D.
Nancy L. Weigel, Ph.D.

Ben-Gurion University of the Negev (Israel)
$375,000
Ron N. Apte, Ph.D.
Joseph Levy, Ph.D.
Angel Porgador, Ph.D.
Shraga Segal, Ph.D.

Brandeis University
$250,000
Lizbeth Hedstrom, Ph.D.
Gregory A. Petsko, Ph.D.

Burnham Institute
$1,786,000
Wadih Arap, M.D., Ph.D.
Nuria E. Assa-Munt, Ph.D.
Kathryn R. Ely, Ph.D.
John C. Reed, M.D., Ph.D.
Erkki Ruoslahti, M.D., Ph.D.

California Institute of Technology
$450,000
Raymond J. Deshaies, Ph.D.
Huatao Guo, Ph.D.
Alexander J. Varshavsky, Ph.D.

California Pacific Medical Center
$100,000
Robert J. Debs, M.D.

Cancer Institute of New Jersey
$75,000
Robert S. DiPaola, M.D.

Cantonal Hospital St. Gall (Switzerland)
$75,000
Marcus Groettrup, Ph.D.

Case Western Reserve University

$350,000
Sanford Markowitz, M.D., Ph.D.
Bingcheng Wang, Ph.D.

Cedars-Sinai Medical Center

$2,095,000
David B. Agus, M.D.
H. Phillip Koeffler, M.D.
Isett Laux, Ph.D.

Cleveland Clinic Foundation

$150,000
Katerina Gurova, Ph.D.
Edward Plow, Ph.D.

Cold Spring Harbor Laboratory

$100,000
Robert Lucito, Ph.D.

Columbia University

$2,129,500

Allen Pavilion Presbyterian Hospital

Carl A. Olsson, M.D.

Atchley Pavilion

Ralph Buttyan, Ph.D.

College of Physicians and Surgeons

Paul B. Fisher, Ph.D.
Aaron E. Katz, M.D.
Nickolas Papadopoulos, Ph.D.

Columbia Presbyterian Medical Center

Daniel Petrylak, M.D.

Cornell University

$4,100,000
Beatrice S. Knudsen, M.D., Ph.D
David M. Nanus, M.D.

New York Presbyterian Hospital

Neil H. Bander, M.D.

Dartmouth-Hitchcock Medical Center

$75,000
Marc S. Ernstoff, M.D.

Duke University

$975,000
Eli Gilboa, Ph.D.
Susan Halabi, Ph.D.
Michael C. Pirrung, Ph.D.
David T. Price, M.D.
Johannes W. Vieweg, M.D.

Eastern Virginia Medical School

$175,000
George L. Wright Jr., Ph.D.

Emory University

$250,000
Wayne Harris, M.D.
John A. Petros, M.D.

Erasmus University (Netherlands)

$250,000
Jan Trapman, Ph.D.
Gert J. van Steenbrugge, Ph.D.

Fred C. Hutchinson Cancer Research Center

$2,680,000
Peter S. Nelson, M.D.
Elaine A. Ostrander, Ph.D.
Janet L. Stanford, Ph.D.

Georgetown University

$1,000,000

Lombardi Cancer Center

Robert L. Martuza, M.D.
Renxiao Wang, Ph.D.
Shaomeng Wang, Ph.D.
Edward P. Gelmann, M.D.

Hadassah University (Israel)

$425,000
Rachel Bar-Shavit, Ph.D.
Eithan Galun, M.D., Ph.D.
Amnon Peled, Ph.D.
Eli Pikarsky, M.D., Ph.D.
Israel Vlodavsky, Ph.D.

Harvard University

$11,100,000

Beth Israel Deaconess Medical Center

Lewis C. Cantley, Ph.D.
John V. Fragioni, M.D., Ph.D.
Sandra M. Gaston, Ph.D.
Richard Junghans, M.D., Ph.D.
Towia A. Libermann, Ph.D.
Massimo Loda, M.D.
Jan E. Schnitzer, M.D.

Brigham and Women's Hospital

Anthony V. D'Amico, M.D., Ph.D.
Phillip Febbo, M.D.
James W. Fett, Ph.D.
Joshua LaBaer, M.D., Ph.D.
Kevin R. Loughlin, M.D.
Karen A. Olson, Ph.D.
Jeffrey L. Sklar, M.D., Ph.D.

Children's Hospital

Judah Folkman,M.D.
Michael Klagsburn, Ph.D.
Calvin J. Kuo, M.D.
Marsha A. Moses, Ph.D.
Richard C. Mulligan, Ph.D.
Bruce R. Zetter, Ph.D.

Dana-Farber Cancer Institute

Ranaan Berger, M.D., Ph.D.
Myles A. Brown, M.D.
Harvey Cantor, M.D.
Diego Castrillon, M.D., Ph.D
Lan Bo Chen, Ph.D.
Glenn Dranoff, M.D.
Phillip Febbo, M.D.
Daniel J. George, M.D.
William C. Hahn, M.D., Ph.D.
Philip W. Kantoff, M.D.
David M. Livingston, M.D.
Massimo Loda, M.D.
Thomas Roberts, Ph.D.
William R. Sellers, M.D.
Sabina Signoretti, M.D.
Bruce M. Spiegelman, Ph.D.
Robert H. Vonderheide, M.D., D.Phil.

Harvard School of Public Health

June M. Chan, Sc.D.
Edward Giovannucci, M.D.
Laurie H. Glimcher, M.D.
Dimitrios Trichopoulos, M.D.

Massachusetts General Hospital

Joel Finkelstein, M.D.
Robert L. Martuza, M.D.
Matthew R. Smith, M.D., Ph.D.
Ching-Hsuan Tung, Ph.D.
Anthony L. Zietman, M.D.

Hebrew University (Israel)

$800,000
Yinon Ben-Neriah, M.D., Ph.D.
Howard Cedar, M.D., Ph.D.
Eli Keshet, Ph.D.
Alexander Levitzki, Ph.D.
David Naor, Ph.D.

Indiana University

$200,000
Thomas A. Gardner, M.D.
George W. Sledge, M.D.

Institute for Systems Biology

$500,000
Leroy E. Hood, M.D., Ph.D.

John Wayne Cancer Institute

$50,000
Frederick R. Singer, M.D.

Johns Hopkins University

$13,297,000
Philip A. Beachy, Ph.D.
David Berman, M.D., Ph.D.
G. Steven Bova, M.D.
Michael A. Carducci, M.D.
Angelo DeMarzo, M.D., Ph.D.
Samuel R. Denmeade, M.D.
Mario Eisenberger, M.D.
John T. Isaacs, Ph.D.
William B. Isaacs, Ph.D.
Hyam I. Levitsky, M.D.
Joel B. Nelson, M.D.
William G. Nelson, M.D., Ph.D.
Alan W. Partin, M.D., Ph.D.
Ronald Rodriguez, M.D., Ph.D.
Jonathan W. Simons, M.D.
Patrick C. Walsh, M.D.

Karolinska Institute (Sweden)

$75,000
Hans-Olov Adami, M.D., Ph.D.

Klinikum de Justus-Liebig Universitat Giessen (Germany)

$175,000

Trinad Chakraborty

La Jolla Institute for Allergy and Immunology

$75,000

Stephen Schoenberger, Ph.D.

Long Island College Hospital

$15,000

Ivan Grunberger, M.D.

Loyola University Medical Center

$200,000

Eugene D. Kwon, M.D.

McGill University

$75,000

Nahum Sonenberg, Ph.D.

Massachusetts Institute of Technology

$1,535,000

Sandra M. Gaston, Ph.D.
Richard O. Hynes, Ph.D.
Jun Liu, Ph.D.
Peter H. Seeberger, Ph.D.
Ganesh Venkataraman, Ph.D.

Whitehead Institute for Biomedical Research

John M. Essigmann, Ph.D.
Eric S. Lander, Ph.D.
Richard C. Mulligan, Ph.D.

Mayo Clinic and Foundation

$500,000

Lorraine A. Fitzpatrick, M.D.
John C. Morris, M.D.
Donald J. Tindall, Ph.D.

Memorial Sloan-Kettering Cancer Center

$14,335,000

David B. Agus, M.D.
William R. Fair, M.D., F.A.C.S.
George Farmer, Ph.D.
Leonard P. Freedman, Ph.D.

Zvi Fuks, M.D.
Polly Gregor, Ph.D.
Adriana Haimovitz-Friedman, Ph.D.
Warren D.W. Heston, Ph.D.
William Kevin Kelly, M.D.
Philip O. Livingston, M.D.
Paul A. Marks, M.D.
Michael R. McDevitt, Ph.D.
David Nanus, M.D.
Neal Rosen, M.D., Ph.D.
Michael Sadelain, M.D., Ph.D.
Peter T. Scardino, M.D.
David A. Scheinberg, M.D., Ph.D.
Howard I. Scher, M.D
George Sgouros, Ph.D.
David Shaffer, M.D., Ph.D.
Moshe Shike, M.D.
Susan F. Slovin, M.D., Ph.D.
Peter Smith-Jones, Ph.D.
David Solit, M.D.
Jedd D. Wolchok, M.D., Ph.D.

Menzies Centre for Population Health Research (Australia)

$50,000

David A. Mackey, M.D.

Mount Sinai School of Medicine

$275,000

Michael J. Droller, M.D.
Irwin H. Gelman, Ph.D.
John A. Martignetti, M.D., Ph.D.

New York University

$430,000

Maarten C. Bosland, D.V.Sc., Ph.D.
Herbert Lepor, M.D.
Ian J. Mohr, Ph.D.
Samir Taneja, M.D.

Skirball Institute of Biomolecular Medicine

Ruben Abagyan, Ph.D.

Northwest Hospital

$475,000

Gerald P. Murphy, M.D., D.Sc.

Northwestern University

$200,000

Wade Bushman, M.D., Ph.D.
Zhou Wang, Ph.D.

Ohio State University

$100,000

M. Guill Wientjes P h.D.

Oregon Health Sciences University

$100,000

Ron G. Rosenfeld, M.D.

Preventive Medicine Research Institute

$500,000

Dean Ornish, M.D.

Rabin Medical Center (Israel)

$50,000

Avishay Sella, M.D.

Rockefeller University

$500,000

Robert G. Roeder, Ph.D.

Strang Cancer Research Laboratory

Martin Lipkin, M.D.

Salk Institute for Biological Studies

$760,050

Ronald M. Evans, Ph.D.

San Diego Cancer Research

$75,000

R. Michael Williams, M.D., Ph.D.

Scripps Research Institute

$975,000

Ruben A. Abagyan, Ph.D.
K.C. Nicolaou, Ph.D.
Prabhakar Tripuraneni, M.D.

Sheba Medical Center (Israel)

$150,000

Gideon Rechavi, M.D., Ph.D.

Stanford University

$1,225,000

Gerald R. Crabtree, M.D.
David Feldman, M.D.
Calvin J. Kuo, M.D.
John E. McNeal, M.D.
Donna M. Peehl, Ph.D.
Thomas A. Stamey, M.D.

St. Louis University

$75,000

William S.M. Wold, Ph.D.

State University of New York

$112,500

Downstate Medical School

Jack Mydlo, M.D.

Stony Brook

Victor I. Romanov, Ph.D.

Technion, Israel Institute of Technology (Israel)

$625,000

Ami Aronheim, Ph.D.
Aaron Ciechanover, M.D., D.Sc.
Fuad Fares, D.Sc.
Ehud Keinan, Ph.D.
Gera Neufeld, Ph.D.
Israel Vlodavsky, Ph.D.

Tel-Aviv University (Israel)

$400,000

Zvi Fishelson, Ph.D.
Sara Lavi, Ph.D.
Ada Rephaeli, Ph.D.
Ilan Tsarfaty, Ph.D.

Sourasky Medical Center

Ben-Zion Katz, Ph.D.
Avi Orr-Urtreger, M.D., Ph.D.

Thomas Jefferson University

$125,000

Michael J. Mastrangelo, M.D.
Albert J. Wong, M.D.

Tulane University

$500,000

Andrew V. Schally, M.D., Ph.D.

University Hospital, Nijmegen (Netherlands)

$275,000

Marion J.G. Bussemakers, Ph.D.

University of Alabama, Birmingham

$100,000

David T. Curiel, M.D.

University of Arizona

$150,000

Leslie Gunatilaka, Ph.D., B.S.
Mark W. Kunkel, Ph.D.

University of Basel (Switzerland)

$75,000

Lukas Bubendorf, M.D.

University of Bern (Switzerland)

$100,000

George N. Thalmann, M.D.

University of California

$16,790,068

Lawrence Livermore National Laboratory

Christine Hartmann Siantar, Ph.D.

University of California, Berkeley

James P. Allison, Ph.D.
Carolyn Bertozzi, Ph.D.
Arthur A. Hurwitz, Ph.D.
David H. Raulet, Ph.D., B.S.
Peter G. Schultz, Ph.D.
David E. Wemmer, Ph.D.

University of California, Davis

Shing-Jien Kung, Ph.D.

University of California, Los Angeles

Arie S. Belldegrun, M.D.
Michael F. Carey, Ph.D.
Rowan T. Chlebowski, M.D., Ph.D.
Pinchas Cohen, M.D.

Jean B. deKernion, M.D.
Purnima Dubey, Ph.D.
Sanjiv S. Gambhir, M.D., Ph.D.
David Heber, M.D., Ph.D.
Harvey R. Herschman, Ph.D.
Jay R. Lieberman, M.D.
Carl W. Miller, Ph.D.
Ayyappan K. Rajasekaran, Ph.D.
Robert Reiter, M.D.
Peter Rosen, M.D.
Marc A. Seltzer, M.D.
Kathleen M. Sakamoto, M.D.
Charles L. Sawyers, M.D
Marc A. Seltzer, M.D.
Ke Shuai, Ph.D.
Peter Tontonoz, M.D., Ph.D.
Owen N. Witte, M.D.
Hong Wu, M.D., Ph.D.

University of California, San Diego

Dennis A. Carson, M.D.
Randolph D. Christen, M.D.
Lawrence S.B. Goldstein, Ph.D.
Michael G. Rosenfeld, Ph.D.
Helen P. Tighe, Ph.D.
Maurizio Zanetti, M.D.

University of California, San Francisco

Jeffrey Arbeit, M.D.
Allan Balmain, Ph.D.
Elizabeth Blackburn, Ph.D.
Peter R. Carroll, M.D.
June Chan, Sc.D.
Colin C. Collins, Ph.D.
Marc Diamond, M.D.
Robert Fletterick, Ph.D.
Mark W. Frohlich, M.D.
Rodney Kiplan Guy, Ph.D.
Douglas Hanahan, Ph.D.
Ronald H. Jensen, Ph.D.
John Kurhanewicz, Ph.D.
James D. Marks, M.D., Ph.D.
Dean Ornish, M.D.
Mack Roach, III, M.D.
Eric J. Small, M.D.
Thea Tlsty, Ph.D.

University of California, Santa Barbara

Dulal Panda, Ph.D.

University of Chicago

$425,000
Douglas K. Bishop, Ph.D.
Carrie W. Rinker-Schaeffer, Ph.D.
Mitchell H. Sokoloff, M.D.

Ben May Institute for Cancer Research
Shutsung Liao, Ph.D.

University of Colorado

$730,000
L. Michael Glode, M.D.
William E. Huffer, M.D.
Andrew S. Kraft, M.D.
Gary J. Miller, M.D., Ph.D.

University of Connecticut

$100,000
Pramod Srivastava, Ph.D.

University of Edinburgh (Scotland)

$75,000
Fouad K. Habib, Ph.D.

University of Helsinki (Finland)

$200,000

Institute of Biomedicine
Olli A. Janne, M.D., Ph.D.

University of Illinois

$50,000
Nissum Hay, Ph.D.

University of Innsbruck (Austria)

$100,000
Zoran Culig, M.D.

University of Iowa

$75,000
George Weiner, M.D.

University of Kentucky

$100,000
Vivek M. Rangnekar, Ph.D.

University of Maryland

$100,000
Natasha Kyprianou, Ph.D.

University of Massachusetts

$325,000
Michael R. Green, M.D., Ph.D.
Shuk-Mei Ho, Ph.D.
Mani Menon, M.D.

University of Michigan

$3,200,000
Arul M. Chinnaiyan, M.D., Ph.D.
Mark Day, Ph.D.
Evan T. Keller, D.V.M., Ph.D.
Donna Livant, Ph.D.
Kenneth J. Pienta, M.D.
Martin G. Sanda, M.D.
Shaomeng Wang, Ph.D.

University of Munich (Germany)

$100,000
Bernd Gansbacher, M.D.

University of Nebraska, Omaha

$100,000
Ming-Fong Lin, Ph.D.

University of North Carolina, Chapel Hill

$250,000
David Ornstein, M.D.
Terry Van Dyke, Ph.D.

University of Pennsylvania

$400,000
Mark I. Greene, M.D., Ph.D.

Wistar Institute
George C. Prendergast, Ph.D.

University of Pittsburgh

$2,275,000
Michael J. Becich, M.D., Ph.D
Barbara A. Foster, Ph.D
John Gilbertson, M.D.
Susan L. Greenspan, M.D.
Candace S. Johnson, Ph.D.
Joel B. Nelson, M.D.
Donald L. Trump, M.D.
Janey Whalen, Ph.D.

University of Rochester

$400,000

Chawnshang Chang, Ph.D.
Edward Messing, M.D.

University of Southern California

$200,000

Gerhard A. Coetzee, Ph.D.
Donald G. Skinner, M.D.

University of Tampere (Finland)

$300,000

Tapio Visakorpi, M.D., Ph.D.

University of Tennessee

$150,000

Jeffrey Gingrich, M.D.

University of Texas

$10,992,000

Health Science Center at San Antonio

Susan Padalecki, Ph.D.

The M.D. Anderson Cancer Center

Wadih Arap, M.D., Ph.D.
Danai Daliani, M.D.
John DiGiovanni, Ph.D.
Isaiah J. Fidler, D.V.M., Ph.D.
Sue-Hwa Lin, Ph.D.
Christopher J. Logothetis, M.D.
David J. McConkey, Ph.D.
Timothy J. McDonnell, M.D., Ph.D.
Nora M. Navone, M.D., Ph.D.
Christos N. Papandreou, M.D., Ph.D.
Andrew C. von Eschenbach, M.D.
Christopher G. Wood, M.D.

Southwestern Medical Center, Dallas

Jerry W. Shay, Ph.D.

University of Toronto (Canada)

$350,000

Sunnybrook Health Science Center

Shoukat Dedhar, Ph.D.
Robert S. Kerbel, Ph.D.

University of Utah, Health Sciences Center

$100,000

Arthur R. Brothman, Ph.D.

University of Virginia

$3,725,000

Leland W.K. Chung, Ph.D.
Thomas A. Gardner, M.D.
Theresa Guise, M.D.
Deborah Lannigan, Ph.D.
Charles E. Myers, Jr., M.D.
J. Thomas Parsons, Ph.D.
Fraydoon Rastinejad, Ph.D.
Mitchell Sokoloff, M.D.
Michael J. Weber, Ph.D.

University of Washington

$7,873,220

Arthur Camerman, Ph.D.
Martin A. Cheever, M.D.
Leroy Hood, M.D., Ph.D.
Gail Jarvik, M.D., Ph.D.
Paul H. Lange, M.D.
Alvin Liu, Ph.D.
Robert L. Vessella, Ph.D.

University of Wisconsin

$4,075,000

David A. Boothman, Ph.D.
Chawnshang Chang, Ph.D.
David F. Jarrard, M.D.
Douglas G. McNeel, M.D., Ph.D.
George Wilding, M.D.
Donald T. Witiak, Ph.D.

Urological Sciences
Research Foundation

$100,000
Leonard S. Marks, M.D.

Utah State Cancer Registry

$183,420
Janet Stanford, M.D.

Vancouver General Hospital (Canada)

$100,000
Martin Gleave, M.D.

Vanderbilt University

$350,000
Sam Chang, M.D.
Robert Matusik, Ph.D.
Joseph A. Smith, Jr., M.D.

Veteran's Administration

$4,622
Patricia Cornett, M.D.

Volcani Center (Israel)

$180,000
Mark Pines, Ph.D.

Walter Reed Army Medical Center

$50,000
David G. McLeod, M.D., J.D.

Washington University

$3,439,166
William J. Catalona, M.D.
Mark L. Day, Ph.D.
Helen Donis-Keller, Ph.D.
Steven F. Dowdy, Ph.D.
Peter A. Humphrey, M.D., Ph.D.
Jeffrey Milbrandt, M.D., Ph.D.
Nobuyuki Oyama, M.D., Ph.D.
Timothy L. Ratliff, Ph.D.
Brian K. Suarez, Ph.D.

Wayne State University

$350,000
Michael L. Cher, M.D.
Keneth V. Honn, Ph.D.

Harper Hospital

J. Edson Pontes, M.D.

Weizmann Institute of Science (Israel)

$1,625,000
Avri Ben-Ze'ev, Ph.D.
Hadassa Degani, Ph.D.
Zelig Eshhar, Ph.D.
Benjamin Geiger, Ph.D.
Yitzhak Koch, Ph.D.
Yoram Salomon, Ph.D.
Rony Seger, Ph.D.
Yechiel Shai, Ph.D
Yosef Shaul, Ph.D.
David Wallach, Ph.D.
Yosef Yarden, Ph.D.
Yehiel Zick, Ph.D.

Yale University

$200,000
Craig M. Crews, Ph.D.

Rethinking the War on Cancer
Moving from a War of Attrition to a Plan of Attack

Remarks by Michael Milken
Founder and Chairman, The Prostate Cancer Foundation

National Cancer Summit
Washington, D.C., November 14, 1995

In 1971, long before there was MTV, CNN or cellular telephones and when I was still the young head of a research department in New York, Texas Instruments was developing the first pocket calculator. Intel introduced the microchip. And the President of the United States in a speech to the American people declared war on cancer. He promised a cure within the decade.

By 1976, five years later, the "Viking I" spacecraft had beamed back detailed pictures of Mars' desert-like terrain. A team at the Massachusetts Institute of Technology announced the synthesis of a functioning gene. And as the war on cancer neared the promised halfway point, my father was diagnosed with what proved to be a fatal case of malignant melanoma.

By 1993, 22 years had passed and personal computers were in 31 million American homes, 58 million households were wired for cable, and 15 million Americans had become regular users of the Internet. It was also the year that scientists discovered the gene suspected of causing Lou Gehrig's disease. By 1993, the President's promised "cancer cure" deadline was 12 years overdue even though each of the five subsequent U.S. presidents had reaffirmed the war on cancer and six more of my relatives had died from it. Nineteen ninety-three was also the year that I was diagnosed with advanced prostate cancer, a disease for which there is still no cure.

By 1995, 25 years since the war on cancer was declared, PowerBooks have made those first Texas Instrument calculators seem like relics and silicon chips drive everything from microwave ovens to missiles. Yet victory still eludes us in our efforts to find a cure for cancer. In 1971, 335,000 Americans died of the disease. This year, that number will climb to 547,000 — nearly as many Americans as have lost their lives fighting for this country in this century.

And the numbers continue to climb. One in three American families will be touched by cancer, and one out of five babies born in the United States today will someday die of the disease — a greater risk than was faced by our parents or grandparents. Ten million Americans have lost their lives to this disease since the War on Cancer was declared. No one is immune. Not one of the most powerful men in the world — President Bill Clinton — nor one of the world's wealthiest and most successful entrepreneurs — Bill Gates of Microsoft. Sadly, both these men recently lost their mothers to cancer.

Clearly, we have not mobilized all possible resources to win the war on cancer. On the eve of the 25th anniversary of that war, we are in danger of snatching defeat from the jaws of victory by becoming fatigued, unfocused and complacent. It is as if we've accelerated to the top of the mountain, and instead of letting scientific momentum push us forward, we have put our foot on the brake. Today we run the risk of rolling backward and losing valuable ground that could take a generation to make up.

Recently proposed reductions in research by both the public and private sectors threaten to stall the efforts of scientists who have tried to apply to cancer the same ingenuity as we saw them depicted as using in the film, "Apollo 13." The war against cancer, like the effort to rescue the hobbled Apollo 13, is a race against the clock — a race that, ironically, one of those Apollo 13 astronauts ultimately lost in his own fight against the disease. The choice is ours: We can sit back and wait for a cure in a generation or two, losing at least another 10 to 20 million more

American mothers, fathers, children, co-workers and friends. Or we can mobilize and find a cure now.

It is time to rethink the War on Cancer, moving from a war of attrition to a new plan of attack. Due to changes in government funding and the new realities of healthcare economics, we must rethink the strategies of financing the war on cancer and how to execute our offensive. The solution lies in a committed and sustained international mobilization. Cancer is not just an American problem; it's worldwide. Financial and human capital from around the world needs to be mobilized. At the same time, we must dramatically expand the level of private sector involvement, including support from communications and technology companies to create "virtual laboratories" that will enable researchers to collaborate and pool their resources without wasteful duplication of time and effort.

The United States has successfully led and participated in previous international mobilizations. Seven critical elements are required: leadership, communications, collaboration, technology, financial resources, human capital, and most of all, *the will to win*. The most recent example of such a convergence came during the 1991 Gulf War. The success of that effort provides 10 road signs we might follow in re-thinking the war on cancer:

1. **Internationalize the War on Cancer:** Over the last several generations, the United States has led the world in medical research, treatment and scientific innovation. Today, cancer patients from around the world travel to the United States for its superior research and treatment. It represents one of the most unappreciated crown jewels of the American economy and has an immeasurable positive influence on our balance of payments. Nevertheless, our medical research infrastructure is now in danger of weakening from the weight of neglect and lack of sufficient funding. Recent reductions by both the public and private sectors make it all but impossible to sustain even current research efforts. Moreover, it moves us no closer to what I believe is the more realistic minimum $20 billion annual investment that is needed

to deploy the technological and human resources necessary to finally bring the war on cancer to an immediate end.

While this amount is nearly 10 times more than the National Cancer Institute's current $2.2 billion budget, it pales in comparison to the $61.1 billion the nations of the world allocated to win the Gulf War. This international collaboration resulted in the United States contributing less than 15 percent of the direct costs, as opposed to the more than 90 percent it contributes to worldwide cancer research. In the Gulf War, some of the other major contributors included Saudi Arabia and Kuwait ($16 billion each), Japan ($10 billion), Germany ($6.5 billion), United Arab Emirates ($4 billion) and South Korea ($355 million). Moreover, 50 different nations combined their efforts under American leadership in the Gulf War, with 39 countries contributing human resources in the form of troops and support personnel. The total spent for the eight-month military effort is more than twice as much as the roughly $30 billion that the nations of the world have dedicated to the war on cancer over the past quarter-century.

The same international commitment is needed in the war on cancer. Today, more than 90 percent of all cancer deaths occur outside the United States, and rates continue to soar particularly in industrialized nations. Yet we have not succeeded in drafting other nations in this battle. Indeed, other governments have made a relatively small investment on scientific and clinical cancer research. Japan, for example, with the world's second largest economy, currently plans to spend only $543 million on cancer research over 10 years, less than 3 percent of the United States' estimated commitment.

This is not just an American race against cancer. It must involve the entire human race.

2. Investing in the War on Cancer Makes Economic Sense: In the early 1980s, Lee Iacocca came to me with a problem: Every automobile manufactured by Chrysler contained more in medical costs than it did in steel. Iacocca needed an innovative healthcare cost-cutting solution. We found it by helping to build a company called Medco Containment, which was established under the leadership of Marty Wygod. Medco's mission was to reduce healthcare expenses by improving the management of an individual's prescription drug needs. Through the use of national pharmacies, generic drugs and other programs, the company was able to deliver prescriptions at a fraction of the cost. The result was billions of dollars in annual savings to patients, governments and companies like Chrysler. And for Medco's investors, our $30 million initial investment in 1983 grew to $6.6 billion when the company was sold to Merck a decade later.

Time-efficient and cost-effective health delivery systems are just two ways to reduce medical costs. Another way is through increased investments in medical research, which will become even more critical with our aging population. Today, the fastest-growing segment of the U.S. population is Americans over the age of 85; the second-fastest are those over the age of 75. Since 1960, the nation has grown by 60 million people — almost all of them over the age of 18. Whereas one out of every three Americans used to be under the age of 18, now it's only one out of four. This demographic shift is also occurring in other countries, such as China, Japan and Mexico. Since most cancers occur in people over the age of 40, the aging of the world's population will inevitably increase cancer healthcare costs.

"Pay now ... or pay more later" was the advertising slogan for an oil filter product. The manufacturer astutely tried to convince consumers to make a relatively small investment in the product now rather than risk a much more expensive outlay later. The same logic can be applied to the war on cancer, particularly as government spending decisions point to reduced funding on an inflation-adjusted basis. While I would be the first to admit that efficiencies can be achieved, it must be with an eye to the long-term: Currently cancer is costing the nation over $100 billion a year in direct and indirect healthcare costs that can only be reduced through cancer prevention, early detection, and discovery of a cure.

Research investments pay. A 10-year, $175-million clinical trial supported by the National Institutes for Health demonstrated that complications of diabetes can be prevented or delayed with tight control of blood glucose levels. A regimen of glucose monitoring and insulin injections administered daily resulted in significant reductions in diabetic retinopathy and a 50 percent reduction in kidney damage. The research revealed that a $1 billion increase in expenditures to prevent or delay diabetic complications can save approximately $8 billion annually in medical costs.

3. Recruit a World-Class Scientific Cancer Team: One of the keys to success in the Gulf War was the ability to dispatch troops already proficient in the use and deployment of modern technology.

The same approach is needed in the war on cancer. It is estimated that fewer than 10 percent of the world's leading chemists, biologists and other scientists have ever worked in the field of cancer. While those working in cancer labs today include many of the most dedicated and productive researchers in science, the fact remains more talent is needed. Too many scientists have been dissuaded by the lack of sustained financial commitments from the public and private sectors. Fit-and-start funding has increasingly made cancer research a low-growth endeavor — not a magnet for the international mobilization required to find a cure.

Winning the war on cancer requires a multidisciplinary approach — and a means to break down the language barrier that exists between the different kinds of scientists critical to the cancer effort. We need mathematicians and their ability to master matters as small as microprocessing and as large as astrophysics. We need physicists and engineers who can develop the sensitive techniques required for making measurements and miniaturizing biological, chemical and detection procedures. We need chemists to help bring new ways to synthesize and analyze the biological molecules of life. We need biologists to bring insights into what has been created through 3.7 billion years of evolution. We need computer scientists to develop the techniques necessary to analyze the massive amounts of information these other scientific disciplines are making available to cancer research. Finally, we need clinicians and patients to apply these laboratory techniques in the real world.

At the same time, we must work to preserve the infrastructure and talent already in place in scientific labs across the world. Recent research-and-development cutbacks by many pharmaceutical companies have already resulted in approximately 100,000 layoffs — with an estimated 200,000 more employees projected to lose their jobs by the end of the decade. We are at risk of dismantling teams of medical researchers who might hold the keys to unlocking the next great medical secret. A potential solution to this dilemma may be the creation of a matching grant program between for-profit companies and government. This would help spread the risks, as well as any future rewards, while at the same time preserving the medical research infrastructure needed to ultimately aid in finding a cure for cancer and other diseases.

4. **Coordinate Worldwide Cancer Resources**: Another strength of the Allied Gulf War effort was the ability to coordinate the resources of different nations toward a common goal. Rather than dispatch 50 different countries on the same mission, creating unnecessary duplication of time and effort, the Allied nations were organized to focus on distinct tasks that added up to a unified and ultimately successful effort.

The war on cancer needs a similar decision-making structure to reduce duplication of effort and cut through fossilized forms and procedures. To be effective, we must link up scientists, clinicians, patients and even laypersons in a "Manhattan Project" set in the information age. But unlike the bricks-and-mortar investments that were made to assemble the hydrogen bomb scientific team all under the same roof, the investments needed for today's war on cancer should be in communications technology. For example, Intel's new "Proserve" system will make it possible for scientists to communicate through full-motion videoconferencing and document-sharing. This type of "virtual laboratory" will foster greater collaboration and reduce duplication of research.

5. Accelerate the Pace of Technology Transfers from Space and Military to Medical Applications: The technological successes that have come from decades of work by government space and military agencies, in cooperation with private enterprise, should now be deployed in the war on cancer. *Let us use the technological advances from the Cold War to help us win the cancer war.*

Movement in that direction has already begun. The Jet Propulsion Laboratory has started to explore ways to use its computing storage and sequencing technology in medical research. Similarly, NASA is developing advanced ultrasound instrumentation that promises to advance space travel as well as provide high-resolution imaging techniques. The outgrowth of this could be applied to breast examinations without the radiation exposure of mammography. In addition, other government agencies — from the Department of Defense to the CIA — have developed computing and imaging technologies that could have applicability to cancer research.

While these efforts are significant, they are not enough. We need to systematically review all the technology that's been developed through decades of public and private investments in the nation's military and space programs. After the technology has been identified, a crash effort must be made to determine which applications can be converted to research.

6. Push the Technological Envelope: We have made great strides in computing speed, storage capacity and sequencing. By one estimate, everything in computing — from memory and size to information processing speed — has doubled every 18 months for the last 30 years. If the same advances had been applied over the last three decades in the American automobile industry, today's Chevy would be the size of a toaster, cost $200, and get 150,000 miles per gallon.

Using computer databasing techniques that did not exist just five years ago, scientists should be creating and analyzing libraries of cancer genes that may well hold the key to determining what differentiates normal cells from malignant ones. No longer do scientists need to study just one gene or one protein at a time. They should be using new technology that makes it possible to look at tens of thousands of genes simultaneously and find out how they differ. They should also be using other new tools, such as the one that enables researchers to take a single drop of blood from a patient, extract a single piece of DNA, and amplify it a million-fold.

At the same time, advanced robotic laboratories should be created around the world to conduct large-scale biorational drug screening operations. Ten million chemical compounds still exist today — more than 10 percent of which are owned by three companies, Merck, Dupont and Eastman Kodak. Yet according to the National Cancer Institute, only an estimated 46,500 compounds have ever been tested against cancer cell lines. For a relatively small $30 million investment, 37 prototypical advanced robotic devices — each costing $800,000 — could test in a single year four times as many compounds against cancer cell lines as have been tested since the start of the war on cancer.

7. **Create a "World Library of Organic Chemicals":** There is no central depository for the 10 million chemical compounds known to be in existence today. In addition, many of those who own the compounds lack the incentive or the financial ability to conduct testing against cancer cell lines. If these methods are allowed to continue, a generation from now only a small fraction of existing compounds will have been tested. That's why action is needed. An international consortium should be formed to facilitate the rapid testing of every known chemical compound against cancer cell lines. To expedite these tests, we can now employ currently existing robotic devices which individually perform 2.5 million tests a year. If discoveries are made, the marketing and/or royalty rights could go back to the owners of the organic chemicals.

8. Accelerate the Approval of New Drugs: The time required to develop a new drug continues to increase. According to the Pharmaceutical Research and Manufacturers of America, the drug development and approval process took 8.1 years on average in the 1960s, 11.6 years in the 1970s, and 14.2 years in the 1980s. Today it takes 14.8 years. If a cure for a particular kind of cancer were discovered tomorrow, under current regulation it might take 10 to 15 years to get it approved for full distribution.

Similarly, the costs of discovering and developing a new drug continue to soar — from $54 million on average in 1976 to $359 million in 1990. The increasing length and cost of drug development represent a rising barrier to innovation — and threaten the United States' leadership role in drug discovery. Rather than draining time and energy pointing fingers at who might be at fault, let us figure out what we can do to get more drugs to patients more quickly.

That was the purpose of a working meeting sponsored by the Prostate Cancer Foundation last July in Washington, D.C. The meeting, led by noted scientist Dr. Louis Lasagna, brought together scientists, activists, cancer research organizations, and government agency representatives including the Food & Drug Administration. The result of the day-long meeting was a "white paper" that recommended, among other things, possible changes in Phase Three trial procedures that could reduce the time and money required for the approval of cancer drugs. Collaborative efforts such as these represent the best hope for future reforms.

In addition, we must do more to encourage companies to allocate resources to research and development for cancer. Extending patent lives is just one step in the direction of fostering greater investments in this area.

9. Develop Strategies to Quickly get Product to the Marketplace: Like a business, our goal should be to quickly get product to the marketplace — to the patients fighting for their lives. Scientists should be spending their time implementing their ideas

— not spending months to years writing grant proposals, and then waiting additional months or years for approval and funding.

At the Prostate Cancer Foundation, we have tried a new approach to the funding of cancer research. Grant applications are restricted to five pages, and approval is granted within 30-45 days. By comparison, the federal grant process requires mountains of paperwork and an approval process that often takes up to 16 months, even for renewal.

After three years, the Prostate Cancer Foundation's fast-track strategy seems to be working. There has been a more than six-fold increase in the number of applications and more than $20 million in grants have been awarded to hundreds of researchers in 22 states, the District of Columbia, Canada, Scotland, Holland and Israel. It is already the world's largest private source of funding for prostate cancer research, eclipsed only by the National Cancer Institute.

10. Mobilize Cancer Patients and Families Around the World: In the Gulf War, more than 800,000 men and women from around the world served on the front. And several million more support personnel provided backup. More than a half-million of the front-line troops were Americans in their late teens or early 20s — vital young adults with 40 or more years in further life expectancy. Yet they answered the call of our nation's leaders to leave their jobs and families and risk their lives for a country and a cause obscure to many of them. More than 350 never made it home.

Today there are an estimated eight million cancer survivors just in America alone — men and women who in many cases have life expectancies measured in months, not years. Many would gladly enlist as foot soldiers in an effort to help cure a disease that in many cases will be genetically passed on to their children and grandchildren.

I am one of those patients. Though my cancer is now in remission, I would gladly participate in clinical drug trials or donate tissue and blood for laboratory study. Most of my fellow cancer survivors need just one thing: Leadership. *They need to be told what they can do.*

In 1961, John F. Kennedy challenged the American people to ask themselves what they could do for their country. Today, eight million cancer survivors in the United States — joined by tens of millions other survivors from around the world — are asking what we can do to help save our own lives and those of future generations.

Since the war on cancer was declared, there have been six U.S. Presidents, five Speakers of the House, and six Senate Majority Leaders. Each has been well-intentioned in helping lead the war on cancer, but the leadership has not been sustained steadily over time. The American people would not and should not stand for a military war to drag on for 25 years and claim more than 10 million American lives. Yet despite growing fatalities and demoralization of our troops, the war on cancer has been allowed to drift. It's time for real leadership from both the President and Congress.

There will be those who say we must practice patience — that we still lack the information to mount an effective offensive against cancer. But anyone ever involved in war knows that great costs can result from further delay. A very wise military leader recently put it to me this way: "There always comes a time when you must get on with the battle. You cannot sit back and do nothing, because you'll never have perfect intelligence on the enemy. Base your battle plan on the best information you have and be ready to modify your strategy and line of attack. The important thing is just to get on with it."

That military leader is General H. Norman Schwarzkopf, commander of our allied forces in the Gulf War. As a fellow prostate cancer patient, General Schwarzkopf also believes this military lesson should be applied to the war on cancer. The fact is, we have plenty of information to wage our offensive. What we need now is an international mobilization to finally get the job done.

At the very least, we owe this not only to ourselves ... but to our families and our future generations.

We have strived to leave our children a world devoid of war, yet more American lives will be lost in one year to cancer than were lost in all the wars of this century.

We have strived to leave our children with a country free from debt, yet we are burdening them with massive medical costs associated with an aging population and ever-increasing rates of cancer.

We have strived to leave our children with a world that celebrates and cherishes the sanctity of a single human life, yet we are unwilling to make the financial and moral commitments necessary to lift the burden of cancer from the next generation.

Through sins of omission as well as commission, we have created a world where one in five will have their lives cut short by cancer. This is too great a burden to leave to our children and grandchildren.

For those children and the children of future generations, let us find a cure for cancer. Let us do it now.

Let us choose life.

Milken Family Foundation
Cancer Research Awards

The Milken Family Foundation, which was established in 1982 to formalize the philanthropy of Michael and Lowell Milken, has supported a broad range of medical research. One of its programs, the Cancer Research Awards (see Chapter 3), provided individual grants ranging in value from $50,000 to $250,000. The listing below indicates the institutional affiliations of the winners at the time they earned their awards.

Stuart A. Aaronson, M.D.
National Cancer Institute

Thaddeus P. Dryja, M.D.
Massachusetts Eye and Ear Infirmary

Lawrence H. Einhorn, M.D.
Indiana University

Bernard Fisher, M.D.
University of Pittsburgh

Michael M. Gottesman, M.D.
National Cancer Institute

Edward Everett Harlow Jr., M.D.
Harvard Medical School

James F. Holland, M.D.
Mt. Sinai School of Medicine

Wuan Ki Hong, M.D.
M.D. Anderson Cancer Center

Stephen B. Howell, M.D.
University of California, San Diego

Philip Leder, M.D.
Harvard Medical School

Victor Ling, Ph.D.
Ontario Cancer Institute, University of Toronto

Lance A. Liotta, M.D., Ph.D.
National Cancer Institute

John D. Minna, M.D.
National Cancer Institute

Charles Myers, M.D.
National Cancer Institute

Robert F. Ozols, M.D., Ph.D.
Fox Chase Cancer Center

Steven Rosenberg, M.D., Ph.D.
National Cancer Institute

Charles J. Scherr, M.D., Ph.D.
St. Jude Children's Hosptital

Dennis Slamon, M.D., Ph.D.
University of California, Los Angeles

Robert Tijan, Ph.D.
University of California, Berkeley

Bert Vogelstein, M.D.
Johns Hopkins University

Thomas Alexander Waldmann, M.D.
National Cancer Institute

Robert A. Weinberg, Ph.D.
Massachusetts Institute of Technology

Owen N. Witte, M.D.
University of California, Los Angeles

Ernst L. Wynder, M.D.
Memorial Sloan-Kettering Cancer Center

Speakers and Presenters at
PCF Scientific Retreats
1994-2003

Abagyan, Ruben A., Ph.D.
(1999)

Abrams, Paul G., M.D.
(2000)

Adams, Julian, Ph.D.
(2000, 2002, 2003)

Afar, Danny, Ph.D.
(1999)

Agus, David B., M.D.
(1999, 2000, 2001, 2002, 2003)

Allison, James P., Ph.D.
(1998, 1999, 2000, 2001, 2002)

Altschul, Arthur
(1994)

Alvarez, Vernon, Ph.D.
(1994)

Ando, Dale, M.D.
(1999, 2000, 2001)

Apte, Ron N., Ph.D.
(2001)

Arap, Wadih, M.D., Ph.D.
(1998, 1999, 2001)

Ascione, Richard, Ph.D.
(1999, 2000)

Attar, Ricardo, Ph.D.
(1999)

Ayala, Gustavo, M.D.
(2000, 2001)

Babish, John, Ph.D.
(1996)

Balk, Steven P., M.D., Ph.D.
(2000)

Banchereau, Jacques F., Ph.D.
(1998, 1999)

Bander, Neil H., M.D.
(1994, 1995, 1996, 1997, 1998, 1999,   2000, 2001, 2002)

Barkas, Alexander, Ph.D.
(1994)

Baserga, Renato, M.D.
(1998)

Becich, Michael J., M.D., Ph.D.
(2000)

Becker, Gary, Ph.D.
(2002)

Beer, Tomasz M., M.D.
(2001, 2002)

Belldegrun, Arie, M.D.
(1996, 1997)

Benaron, David, M.D.
(2000)

Berg, William J., M.D.
(2002, 2003)

Bergers, Gabriele, Ph.D.
(1998)

Berman, David, M.D., Ph.D.
(2000, 2001)

Bishop, Charles W., Ph.D.
(1999)

Bishop, Douglas K., Ph.D.
(2000)

Bookstein, Robert, M.D.
(1995, 1996)

Boothman, David A., Ph.D.
(1997)

Botstein, David , Ph.D.
(2002)

Bova, G. Steven, M.D.
(1995, 1996, 1997, 1998, 1999)

Boynton, Alton L., Ph.D.
(1996, 1998, 2000, 2001)

Bradley, Matthews O., Ph.D.
(1999, 2000, 2001)

Brawer, Michael K., M.D.
(1996)

Breiger, George, M.D.
(1995)

Briggman, Joseph, Ph.D.
(1995, 1996)

Broder, Samuel, M.D.
(1994 Call-to-Action Dinner, 2002)

Brooks, James D., M.D.
(1999)

Brothman, Arthur R., Ph.D.
(1996)

Brown, Myles A., M.D.
(1997)

Bubendorf, Lukas, M.D.
(2000)

Bussemakers, Marion J.G., Ph.D.
(1997, 1998, 1999)

Buttyan, Ralph, Ph.D.
(1995, 1997)

Camerman, Arthur, Ph.D.
(1995)

Campbell, Moray J., Ph.D.
(2001)

Cantor, Harvey, M.D.
(1999, 2000, 2001)

Carducci, Michael A., M.D.
(1998, 1999, 2000, 2001, 2003)

Carey, Michael F., Ph.D.
(1999, 2000, 2001)

Carretta, Robert, M.D.
(1996)

Carson, Dennis A., M.D.
(2001)

Carter, Stephen, M.D.
(2002)

Castrillon, Diego, M.D., Ph.D.
(2001)

Catalona, William J., M.D.
(1996, 1997, 1998, 1999, 2001)

Celis, Esteban, M.D., Ph.D.
(1994)

Chan, June M., Sc.D.
(1998, 1999, 2000, 2001, 2002)

Chan, Wing Kai, FRACP
(2000)

Chang, Chawnshang, Ph.D.
(1995, 1997, 1998, 1999)

Chedid, Marcio, Ph.D.
(1999)

Cheever, Martin A., M.D.
(1996, 1997)

Chen, Junjie, Ph.D.
(1998)

Chen, Lan Bo, Ph.D.
(1994, 1996)

Cher, Michael L., M.D.
(1996, 2000)

Chirgwin, John, Ph.D.
(2001)

Chlebowski, Rowan T., M.D.,
Ph.D.
(1999)

Christen, Randolph D., M.D.
(1996)

Chung, Leland W.K., Ph.D.
(1994, 1995, 1996, 1997, 1998,
2000, 2001)

Ciechanover, Aaron, M.D., D.Sc.
(2002)

Coffey, Donald S., Ph.D.
(1997, 1998, 1999, 2000, 2001,
2002, 2003)

Cohen, Pinchas, M.D.
(2000, 2001)

Cooper, Michael R., M.D.
(2001)

Corey, David, Ph.D.
(1996)

Crabtree, Gerald R., M.D.
(2001)

Cravatt, Ben
(2000)

Crews, Craig M., Ph.D.
(1997, 1998)

Culig, Zoran, M.D.
(1999)

Dalbagni, Guido, M.D.
(1994)

Daliani, Danai, M.D.
(2000, 2001)

D'Amico, Anthony V., M.D.,
Ph.D.
(2000, 2001, 2002, 2003)

Dannull, Jens, Ph.D.
(2000)

Davis, Governor Gray
(2001)

Davis, Tom, M.D.
(2001)

Dawson, Robert, M.D.
(1999)

Day, Mark, Ph.D.
(1994)

Debs, Robert J., M.D.
(1996)

Dedhar, Shoukat, Ph.D.
(1995)

Degani, Hadassa, Ph.D.
(2001)

DeMarzo, Angelo, M.D., Ph.D.
(2001)

Desai, Ashvin, Ph.D.
(1999)

Devi, Gayathri, Ph.D.
(2000, 2001)

Dickey, Robert, IV, Ph.D.
(1999)

DiPaola, Robert S., M.D.
(2000)

Dole, U.S. Senator Bob
(2002)

Donis-Keller, Helen, Ph.D.
(1996)

Donovan, Gerald, Ph.D.
(1999)

Dowdy, Steven F., Ph.D.
(2000)

Drew, Lisa, Ph.D.
(2000)

Dubey, Purnima, Ph.D.
(1999, 2000, 2001)

Ely, Kathryn R., Ph.D.
(1997, 1999, 2000)

Ernstoff, Marc, M.D.
(1995)

Eshhar, Zelig, Ph.D.
(1996, 1999, 2001)

Essigmann, John M., Ph.D.
(1996, 1997, 1998,
1999, 2000, 2001)

Evans, Ronald M., Ph.D.
(1997, 1998, 2001, 2002)

Fair, William R., M.D., FACS
(1994, 1996, 1997)

Fares, Fuad, D.Sc.
(2001)

Farmer, George, Ph.D.
(1999)

Felciano, Ramon, Ph.D.
(2003)

Feldman, David, M.D.
(1995, 2002)

Ferry, Robert J. Jr., M.D.
(1999)

Fett, James W., Ph.D.
(1995, 1999, 2000)

Fidler, Isaiah J., D.V.M., Ph.D.
(1994, 1995 1996, 1997)

Figg, William D., Pharm. D.
(1997)

Fisher, Paul, Ph.D.
(1995, 1996)

Fitzpartrick, Lorraine, M.D.
(1994, 1995)

Fletterick, Robert, Ph.D.
(2003)

Folkman, Judah, M.D.
(1994, 1996, 1998)

Foster, Barbara A., Ph.D.
(2001)

Freeman, Michael, Ph.D.
(1996)

Fritz, Larry, Ph.D.
(1994, 1996)

Fritzberg, Alan R., Ph.D.
(1998)

Frohlich, Mark W., M.D.
(1999, 2000, 2001)

Fuks, Zvi, M.D.
(1997)

Fyfe, Gwen, M.D.
(2001)

Gaeta, Frederico, Ph.D.
(1995)

Gallo, Robert C., M.D.
(1997)

Gambhir, Sanjiv S., M.D., Ph.D.
(1998, 2001, 2002)

Gann, Peter, M.D., Sc.D.
(2003)

Gansbacher, Bernd, M.D.
(1995)

Garcia-Manero, Guillermo, M.D.
(1999)

Gardner, Thomas A., M.D.
(1998, 1999, 2001)

Garzotto, Mark, M.D.
(1997)

Gaston, Sandra M., Ph.D.
(1998, 2000, 2001)

Gelman, Irwin H., Ph.D.
(1998)

Gelmann, Edward P., M.D.
(1994, 1995, 1996,
1997, 2002)

Geltosky, Jack
(1997)

George, Daniel J., M.D.
(2000)

Gilbertson, John, M.D.
(2001)

Gilboa, Eli, Ph.D.
(1994, 1995, 1996)

Gill, Parkash, M.D.
(2000)

Gillis, Steven, Ph.D.
(1995)

Giovannucci, Edward, M.D.
(1999, 2000)

Glimcher, Laurie H., M.D.
(2000, 2001)

Glode, L. Michael, M.D.
(1995, 2001)

Goeckler, William, Ph.D.
(1995, 2003)

Goldberg, Jeremy P.
(1997)

Golde, David W., M.D.
(1999)

Goldstein, Lawrence S.B., Ph.D.
(1997)

Golomb, Eliahu, M.D., Ph.D.
(2000)

Gomella, Leonard, M.D.
(2003)

Gong, Michael C., M.D., Ph.D.
(2000)

Goulet, Robert
(1994 Call-to-Action Dinner)

Graff, Jeremy, Ph.D.
(1999)

Green, Michael R., M.D., Ph.D.
(2000)

Green, Shawn J., Ph.D.
(2000)

Greenberg, Norman M., Ph.D.
(1995, 1996, 1998, 1999,
2000, 2001)

Greene, Mark I., M.D., Ph.D.
(1996)

Gregor, Polly, Ph.D.
(2000, 2001, 2002)

Grossman, Shlomo, Ph.D.
(2001)

Grove, Andrew S., Ph.D.
(1997)

Gubish, Edward R., Ph.D.
(1999)

Gunatilaka, Leslie, Ph.D., B.S.
(2001)

Habib, Fouad, Ph.D.
(1995)

Hahn, William C., M.D., Ph.D.
(2001)

Haimovitz-Friedman, Adriana,
Ph.D.
(1995, 1996, 1998)

Harley, Calvin, Ph.D.
(1994)

Harlow, Edward E., Ph.D.
(1999)

Harris, Wayne B., M.D.
(2001)

Hartmann Siantar, Christine L.,
Ph.D.
(1998, 1999)

Hawkins, Cheryl
(1999)

Healy, Cynthia, Ph.D.
(1994)

Heber, David, M.D., Ph.D.
(1995, 1997, 1998,
1999, 2000, 2001,
2002, 2003)

Hedlund, Jay H.
(1997)

Hedstrom, Lizbeth, Ph.D.
(2003)

Henderson, Daniel, M.D., Ph.D.
(1998, 1999, 2000)

Herlihy, Walter, Ph.D.
(1994)

Herschman, Harvey R., Ph.D.
(1997)

Heston, Warren D.W., Ph.D.
(1995, 1996, 1997,
1998, 1999)

Higano, Celestia S., M.D.
(2001)

Hillman, Robert S.
(2000)

Holaday, John W., Ph.D.
(1999)

Holden, Stuart, M.D.
(1994 Call-to-Action Dinner,
1996, 1997)

Holmes, Edward, M.D.
(2003)

Holroyd, Kenneth J., M.D.,
M.S.B.
(1999)

Hood, Leroy E., M.D., Ph.D.
(1995, 1996, 1997, 1998,
1999, 2000, 2001,
2002, 2003)

Hsieh, Chia-Ling, Ph.D.
(2001)

Huffer, William E., M.D.
(1999)

Humerickhouse, Rod, M.D.,
Ph.D.
(2001)

Humphrey, Peter A., M.D., Ph.D.
(1996, 1998, 2001)

Hurwitz, Arthur A., Ph.D.
(2000)

Hwang, Leon C., M.D.
(1997)

Ide, Hisamitsu, M.D., Ph.D.
(2000, 2001)

Ingber, Donald, M.D., Ph.D.
(1994)

Ingle, Blake, Ph.D.
(1994)

Isaacs, John T., Ph.D.
(1996, 1997, 1998,
1999, 2001)

Isaacs, William B., Ph.D.
(1994, 1995, 1996, 1999)

Israel, Robert J., M.D.
(1999)

Iversen, Patrick, Ph.D.
(1999, 2000)

Jackson, Richard, Ph.D.
(2000, 2001)

Jain, Rakesh, Ph.D.
(1995)

Jakobovits, Aya, Ph.D.
(1999, 2000, 2001)

Janne, Olli A., M.D., Ph.D.
(2000, 2001)

Jehonathan, Pinthus, M.D.
(1997)

Jensen, Ronald, Ph.D.
(1995)

Johnson, Candace S., Ph.D.
(2001)

Jones, Deborah
(2000)

Jones, Raymond
(2000)

Jordan, Hamilton
(2002)

Kadmon, Dov, M.D.
(1994)

Kantoff, Philip W., M.D.
(1997, 2000, 2001)

Kaplan-Lefko, Paula J., Ph.D.
(2001)

Karpf, David B., M.D.
(2000)

Kattan, Michael W., Ph.D.
(2000)

Katz, Aaron E., M.D.
(1997)

Kauffman, Michael G., M.D.,
Ph.D.
(2000, 2001)

Kay, Andrea, M.D.
(2000)

Kelly, William Kevin, M.D.
(2001)

Keoffler, H. Philip, M.D.
(1996)

Kerbel, Robert S., Ph.D.
(1998, 1999, 2000, 2001)

Kessler, David, M.D.
(2002)

Kirschenbaum, Alexander, M.D.
(1994)

Klagsbrun, Michael, Ph.D.
(1998, 2000)

Klausner, Richard, M.D.
(1996, 2000)

Klein, Eric, M.D.
(2003)

Koeffler, H. Phillip, M.D.
(1995, 1996, 1999)

Koeneman, Kenneth S., M.D.
(1999)

Kowal, Charles, M.D.
(1995)

Kraft, Andrew S., M.D.
(1996)

Kumar, Vijay, Ph.D., M.
(1994)

Kuo, Calvin J., M.D., Ph.D.
(2000, 2001)

Kurhanewicz, John, Ph.D.
(1996)

Kwon, Eugene D., M.D.
(2001)

Kylstra, Jelle, M.D.
(2001)

Kyprianou, Natasha, Ph.D.
(1997)

LaBaer, Joshua, M.D., Ph.D.
(2000)

Lamb, Dolores, Ph.D.
(1995)

Lamm, Marilyn, Ph.D.
(2000)

Lander, Eric S., Ph.D.
(1996)

Lange, Paul H., M.D.
(1994, 1995, 1996, 1997,
1998, 2001)

Laxmanan, Seethalakshmi, Ph.D.
(1996)

Lee, David, M.D.
(2003)

Leiden, Jeff, M.D., Ph.D.
(2002)

Levine, Arnold, Ph.D.
(2003)

Levitsky, Hyam, M.D.
(1995, 1996)

Li, Jim
(2000)

Libermann, Towia A., Ph.D.
(1999, 2001)

Lieberman, Jay R., M.D.
(1999, 2000, 2001)

Lieberman, Ron, M.D.
(2000)

Lin, Ming-Fong, Ph.D.
(1995)

Lin, Sue-Hwa, Ph.D.
(1998, 2001)

Linehan, W. Marston, M.D.
(1994)

Liotta, Lance, M.D.
(1997)

Lipkin, Martin, M.D.
(1999)

Liu, Alvin, Ph.D.
(1997, 1998, 1999, 2000,
2001)

Liu, Jun, Ph.D.
(1998)

Livant, Donna, Ph.D.
(2001)

Livingston, Philip O., M.D.
(1996, 1997, 1999)

Loda, Massimo, M.D.
(1996, 1998)

Logothetis, Christopher J., M.D.
(1994, 1995, 1996, 1997,
1998, 1999, 2000, 2001,
2002, 2003)

Lowy, Israel, M.D., Ph.D.
(2003)

Lyerly, H. Kim, M.D.
(1997)

Mack, David H., Ph.D.
(2000)

Mack, David, Ph.D.
(1997)

Maguire, Yu-Ping, Ph.D.
(2000)

Maguire, Robert T., M.D.
(1996)

Marks, James D., M.D., Ph.D.
(1996, 1997)

Marks, Leonard S., M.D.
(2001, 2002)

Martin, Graeme, Ph.D.
(2001)

Martuza, Robert L., M.D.
(1998, 1999, 2000, 2001)

Mascarenhas, Desmond, Ph.D.
(1999, 2000)

Mashal, Robert D., M.D.
(1998, 1999)

Mazar, Andrew P., Ph.D.
(2001, 2003)

McConkey, David J., Ph.D.
(1998)

McCormick, Frank, Ph.D.
(1994)

McDevitt, Michael R., Ph.D.
(2000)

McDonnell, Timothy J., M.D.,
Ph.D.
(1995, 1996, 1997, 1998,
1999)

McGuinn, David, M.S., Ph.D.
(1995)

McLeod, David, M.D., J.D.
(1995)

McMahon, Jerry, Ph.D.
(1994)

McNeal, John E., M.D.
(1997)

Milbrandt, Jeffrey D., M.D.,
Ph.D.
(1996, 1997, 1998, 1999,
2000, 2001, 2003)

Milken, Michael
(1994, 1995, 1996, 1997,
1998, 1999, 2000, 2001,
2002, 2003)

Miller, Carl W., Ph.D.
(2001)

Miller, Gary J., M.D., Ph.D.
(1997, 1998, 2000)

Miller, Governor Bob
(2000)

Misrock, S. Leslie, J.D.
(1996, 1997, 1998)

Mohler, James L., M.D.
(2003)

Mohr, Ian J., Ph.D.
(2000)

Monahan, John, Ph.D.
(1994)

Moorin, Jay
(2003)

Moreno, Jose G., M.D.
(2000, 2001)

Morris, John C., M.D.
(1999)

Morris, Michael J., M.D.
(2001)

Moses, Marsha A., Ph.D.
(1996)

Mueller, Elisabetta, Ph.D.
(1998, 1999)

Mulligan, Richard C., Ph.D.
(1994, 1997)

Murphy, Gerald P., M.D., D.Sc.
(1995, 1997, 1998, 1999)

Myers, Charles E. Jr., M.D.
(1994, 1995, 1996, 1997, 1999,
2000)

Namoto, Kenji
(2000)

Nanus, David M., M.D.
(1996, 1997, 1998, 2000,
2001)

Natale, Ronald, M.D.
(1994)

Nauman, David
(2000)

Navone, Nora M., M.D., Ph.D.
(1997, 1998, 1999, 2000,
2001)

Needleman, Philip
(2002)

Nelson, Barbara
(2001)

Nelson, Joel B., M.D.
(1996, 1997, 1998, 1999,
2000, 2003)

Nelson, Peter S., M.D.
(1997, 1998, 1999, 2000,
2001, 2002)

Nelson, William G., M.D., Ph.D.
(1994, 1996, 1997, 1998,
1999, 2000, 2001, 2002,
2003)

Neubauer, Blake Lee, Ph.D.
(1999, 2000, 2003)

Nicolaou, Kyriacos C., Ph.D.
(1996, 1997)

Nigg, Karl, J.D.
(2000)

Norton, Larry, M.D.
(2003)

Nouri-Shirazi, Mahyar, DVM,
Ph.D.
(2000)

Oliff, Allen, M.D.
(1995)

Olson, William C., Ph.D.
(2000, 2001)

Olumi, Aria F., M.D.
(1998)

O'Malley, Bert W., M.D.
(1998, 1999)

Oren, Moshe, Ph.D.
(2003)

Ornish, Dean M., M.D.
(1997, 1999)

Ornstein, David K., M.D.
(2001)

Oshima, Shin-ichi, M.D., Ph.D.
(1995)

Ostrander, Elaine A., Ph.D.
(1996, 1997, 1998)

Oyama, Nobuyuki, M.D., Ph.D.
(2001)

Pamukcu, Rifat, M.D.
(1999)

Panda, Dulal, Ph.D.
(2000)

Pang, Shen, Ph.D.
(1994)

Panicali, Dennis, Ph.D.
(1995)

Papadopoulos, Nickolas, Ph.D.
(1999)

Papandreou, Christos N., M.D.,
Ph.D.
(1999, 2000, 2001)

Parkinson, David, M.D.
(2002)

Parsons, J. Thomas, Ph.D.
(1997, 1999, 2000, 2001)

Partin, Alan W., M.D., Ph.D.
(1998)

Pazdur, Richard, M.D.
(2002)

Peehl, Donna M., Ph.D.
(1994, 1996, 1997, 1998,
2000, 2001)

Pereira, Fred, Ph.D.
(1997)

Petros, John, M.D.
(1994)

Petrylak, Daniel P., M.D.
(1999, 2000, 2001)

Petsko, Gregory A., D.Phil.
(1998, 1999)

Pettaway, Curtis A., M.D.
(2001)

Phelps, Michael E., Ph.D.
(1996, 2000)

Pienta, Kenneth J., M.D.
(1994, 1995, 1996, 1997,
1998, 1999, 2000)

Pines, Mark, Ph.D.
(2001)

Pirie-Shepherd, Steven, Ph.D.
(1999)

Plow, Edward, Ph.D.
(2000, 2001)

Polascik, Thomas J., M.D.
(1999)

Pollak, Michael N., M.D.
(2001)

Prendergast, George C., Ph.D.
(1997, 1998)

Prentki, Ronald
(1999)

Purvis, Joseph D., M.D.
(2000)

Raffo, Anthony, Ph.D.
(1994)

Ralph, David, Ph.D.
(1997)

Rangnekar, Vivek M., Ph.D.
(1998)

Raschke, William C., Ph.D.
(2001)

Ratliff, Timothy, Ph.D.
(1995, 1996)

Reed, John C., M.D., Ph.D.
(1995, 1996, 1997, 1998,
1999, 2000, 2001, 2002)

Reeders, Stephen T., M.D.
(1996)

Reiser, H. Joseph, Ph.D.
(2000)

Reiter, Robert E., M.D.
(1997, 1998, 1999, 2000,
2001)

Rheinstein, Peter, M.D., J.D.,
M.S.
(2000, 2001)

Rice, Glenn, Ph.D.
(2003)

Richard, Fabian, Ph.D.
(2001)

Richon, Victoria M., Ph.D.
(2001)

Rinker-Schaeffer, Carrie W.,
Ph.D.
(1997)

Rittmaster, Roger, M.D.
(2002)

Roach, Mack III, M.D.
(1998, 2001)

Rodriguez, Ronald, M.D., Ph.D.
(1997, 1999, 2000, 2001)

Roeder, Robert G., Ph.D.
(2000, 2001)

Romanov, Victor I., Ph.D.
(1998, 1999)

Rosania, Gustavo R., Ph.D.
(1998)

Rosen, Neal, M.D., Ph.D.
(1997, 1998, 2000, 2001,
2002, 2003)

Rosenfeld, Michael G., M.D.,
Ph.D.
(1998, 1999, 2000, 2001)

Rosenfeld, Ron G., M.D.
(1999)

Ross, Sara Jane
(2000)

Rote, Bill, Ph.D.
(2000)

Rowley, David R., Ph.D.
(1998)

Ruoslahti, Erkki I., M.D., Ph.D.
(1999)

Ryan, Christopher, M.D.
(2000)

Sacks, Natalie, M.D.
(2003)

Saedi, Mo, Ph.D.
(1998, 1999, 2000, 2001)

Saez, Enrique, Ph.D.
(1999, 2000)

Sakamoto, Kathleen M., M.D.
(2000)

Sanda, Martin G., M.D.
(1997)

Sandler, Howard, M.D.
(2001)

Sasisekharan, Ram, Ph.D.
(1999)

Sawyers, Charles L., M.D.
(1996, 1997, 1998, 1999,
2000, 2001, 2002)

Scardino, Peter T., M.D.
(1996, 1997, 1998, 2000,
2001, 2003)

Schally, Andrew V., M.D., Ph.D.
(1997, 1998, 1999, 2000,
2001)

Scheinberg, David A., M.D.,
Ph.D.
(1997, 1998, 1999)

Schenkein, David, M.D.
(2003)

Scher, Howard I., M.D.
(1994, 1995, 1996, 1997,
1998, 1999, 2000, 2001,
2002, 2003)

Scher, Nancy, M.D.
(1997)

Schlom, Jeffrey, Ph.D.
(1995)

Schnitzer, Jan E., M.D.
(1996, 1997)

Schrader, William, Ph.D.
(1998)

Schreiber, Alain
(1999)

Schwimmer, Judy, M.B.A., M.A.
(1999)

Scott, Randy, Ph.D.
(2001)

Seeberger, Peter H., Ph.D.
(1999, 2000, 2001)

Sella, Avishay, M.D.
(2001)

Sellers, William R., M.D.
(1998, 1999, 2000, 2001,
2003)

Seltzer, Marc A., M.D.
(2000)

Sepp-Lorenzino, Laura, Ph.D.
(1999)

Shaffer, David R., M.D., Ph.D.
(2001)

Shay, Jerry W., Ph.D.
(1996, 2000, 2001)

Shelby, Senator Richard
(1994 Call-to-Action Dinner)

Sherman, Michael I., Ph.D.
(1998)

Shike, Moshe, M.D.
(1998)

Shou, Jianyong, Ph.D.
(2000)

Shtern, Faina, M.D.
(2001)

Shuman, Marc A., M.D.
(2000, 2001)

Shyjan, Andrew, Ph.D.
(1998)

Signorello, Lisa, Sc.D.
(1998)

Silva, John, M.D.
(1999)

Silver, Daniel, M.D., Ph.D.
(1999)

Simon, Mark J.
(1998, 1999, 2000, 2002,
2003)

Simons, Jonathan W., M.D.
(1995, 1996, 1997, 1998,
1999, 2002, 2003)

Singer, Frederick R., M.D.
(1998, 2001)

Singer, Jack W., M.D.
(1999, 2000, 2001)

Sinha, Akhouri A., Ph.D.
(1999, 2000)

Sklar, Jeffrey, M.D., Ph.D.
(1995)

Slamon, Dennis J., M.D., Ph.D.
(1998)

Slater, Eve, M.D.
(2002)

Slovin, Susan Faith, M.D., Ph.D.
(1998, 1999, 2000, 2001)

Small, Eric J., M.D.
(1998, 1999, 2000, 2001,
2002)

Smith, Joseph Jr., M.D.
(1994)

Smith, Matthew R., M.D., Ph.D.
(1999, 2000, 2001, 2002)

Smith, Sanford
(1995)

Sobol, Robert E., M.D.
(1998, 2000)

Sokoloff, Mitchell H., M.D.
(1998, 2000)

Soule, Howard R., Ph.D.
(1997, 1998)

Spitler, Lynn, M.D.
(1994)

Srivastava, Pramod, Ph.D.
(1997)

Stanford, Janet, Ph.D.
(1996, 1997, 1998, 2002)

Stein, Robert, M.D., Ph.D.
(1994, 1995)

Steiner, Mitchell, Ph.D.
(1994, 2003)

Stevens, Senator Ted
(2000)

Suarez, Brian K., Ph.D.
(1996, 1997)

Sun, Leon, M.D., Ph.D.
(2001)

Sweeney, Christopher John,
MBBS
(2000)

Swindell, Charles S., Ph.D.
(2000)

Taneja, Samir S., M.D.
(2001)

Thompson, Timothy C., Ph.D.
(1994, 1995, 1996, 1997,
1998, 1999)

Tighe, Helen, Ph.D.
(1996)

Tontonoz, Peter, M.D., Ph.D.
(2000, 2001)

Trachtenberg, John, M.D.,
FRCS(C)
(2000)

Trapman, Jan, Ph.D.
(1997)

True, Lawrence D., M.D.
(2001)

Trump, Donald L., M.D.
(1994, 1998, 1999, 2000,
2001)

Ts'o, Paul O.P., Ph.D.
(1999)

Valone, Frank, M.D.
(1998, 1999)

Van Steenbrugge, Gert, Ph.D.
(1996)

Varshavsky, Alexander J., Ph.D.
(1996, 1997)

Veltri, Robert, Ph.D.
(1995, 1996, 1998, 1999,
2001)

Vessella, Robert L., Ph.D.
(1996, 1999, 2000)

Vieweg, Johannes W., M.D.
(2000, 2001)

Vigneron, Daniel B., Ph.D.
(1998, 1999, 2000)

Visakorpi, Tapio, M.D., Ph.D.
(1997, 1998, 1999)

von Eschenbach, Andrew C.,
M.D.
(1994, 1995, 1996, 1997,
1998, 2001, 2002, 2003)

Vonderheide, Robert H., M.D.,
D.Phil.
(2000, 2001)

Vourloumis, Dionisios, Ph.D.
(1998)

Wagner, Julie
(2000)

Waksal, M.D., Harlan
(1995, 1996)

Walsh, Patrick C., M.D.
(1995, 1998, 2003)

Wang, Bingcheng, Ph.D.
(2001)

Wang, Shaomeng, Ph.D.
(2001)

Wang, Zhou, Ph.D.
(1997)

Ward, David C., Ph.D.
(1998)

Wasilkenko, William, Ph.D.
(1994, 1995)

Wasserman, William
(1999)

Watabe, Testuro, Ph.D.
(1999)

Webb, Iain J., M.D.
(2003)

Weber, Michael J., Ph.D.
(1997, 1998, 1999, 2000,
2001, 2002)

Webster, Nicholas, Ph.D.
(2001)

Weigel, Nancy L., Ph.D.
(2001)

Weiner, George, M.D.
(1995)

Weinmann, Roberto, Ph.D.
(2001)

West, Michael D., Ph.D.
(1997)

Wick, Michael M., M.D., Ph.D.
(2001)

Wientjes, M. Guill, Ph.D.
(1996)

Wilding, George, M.D.
(1994, 1995, 1996, 1997,
1998, 1999, 2000, 2001,
2002, 2003)

Wilds, Dan
(2000)

Williams, Jon I., Ph.D.
(1998)

Williams, Lewis T., M.D., Ph.D.
(1997)

Wilson, Les, Ph.D.
(2000)

Winters, Barbara
(1994)

Witte, Owen N., M.D.
(1996, 1997, 1999, 2000,
2001, 2003)

Wolchok, Jedd D., M.D., Ph.D.
(2000, 2001)

Wold, William S.M., Ph.D.
(2000)

Wood, Christopher G., M.D.
(1999)

Wood, Christopher, M.D.
(1999)

Wu, Hong, M.D., Ph.D.
(2000, 2001)

Xu, Jiangchun, Ph.D.
(1999)

Yarden, Yosef, Ph.D.
(2003)

Ye, Xiang-cang, Ph.D.
(2000)

Zanetti, Maurizio, M.D.
(2001)

Zeldis, Jerome B., M.D., Ph.D.
(2003)

Zetter, Bruce R., Ph.D.
(1995, 1997)

Zhang, Yingsheng, Ph.D.
(1998)

Zick, Yehiel, Ph.D.
(2001)

Zietman, Anthony, M.D.
(1995)

Zurowski, Vincent, Ph.D.
(1994)

Index of Names